INTIMATE PARTNER VIOLENCE
Escape Room

FROM ABUSE TO FREEDOM, SURVIVORS TELL THEIR STORIES

REBECCA MIGDAL

WITH THE COLLABORATION OF

SADIE ROSE • JENNIE CHI • JASMINE DELUDE • V

© 2019 MYTHOPRINT PUBLISHING

A person from any background can become trapped in a pattern of abuse.

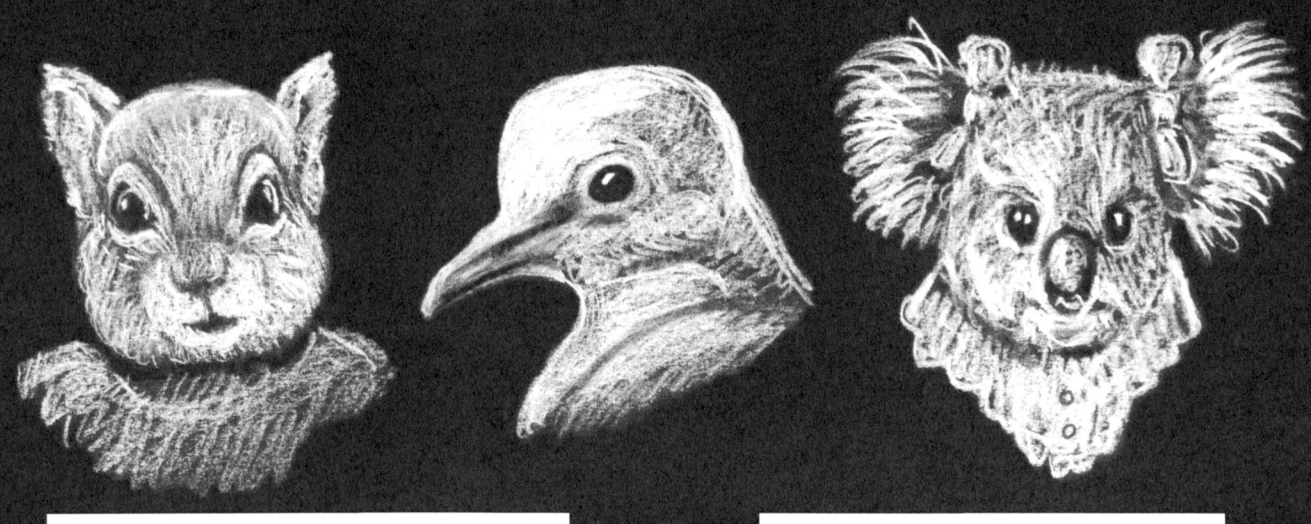

Maybe you're disabled, homeless, mentally ill, or have an addiction...

Maybe you're a doctor, college professor, judge or engineer.

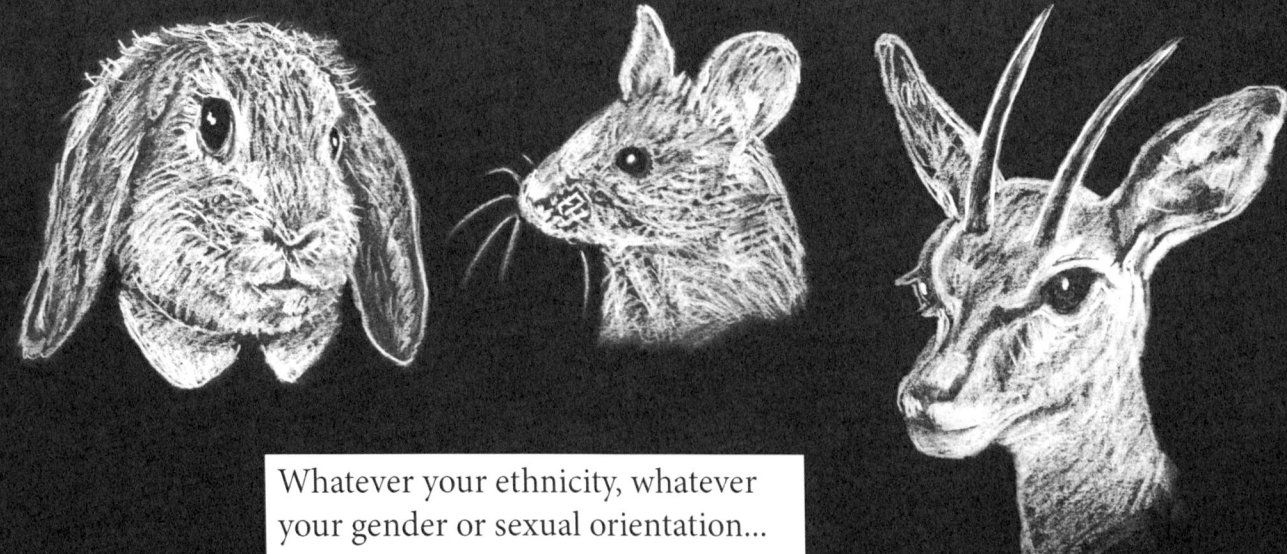

Whatever your ethnicity, whatever your gender or sexual orientation...

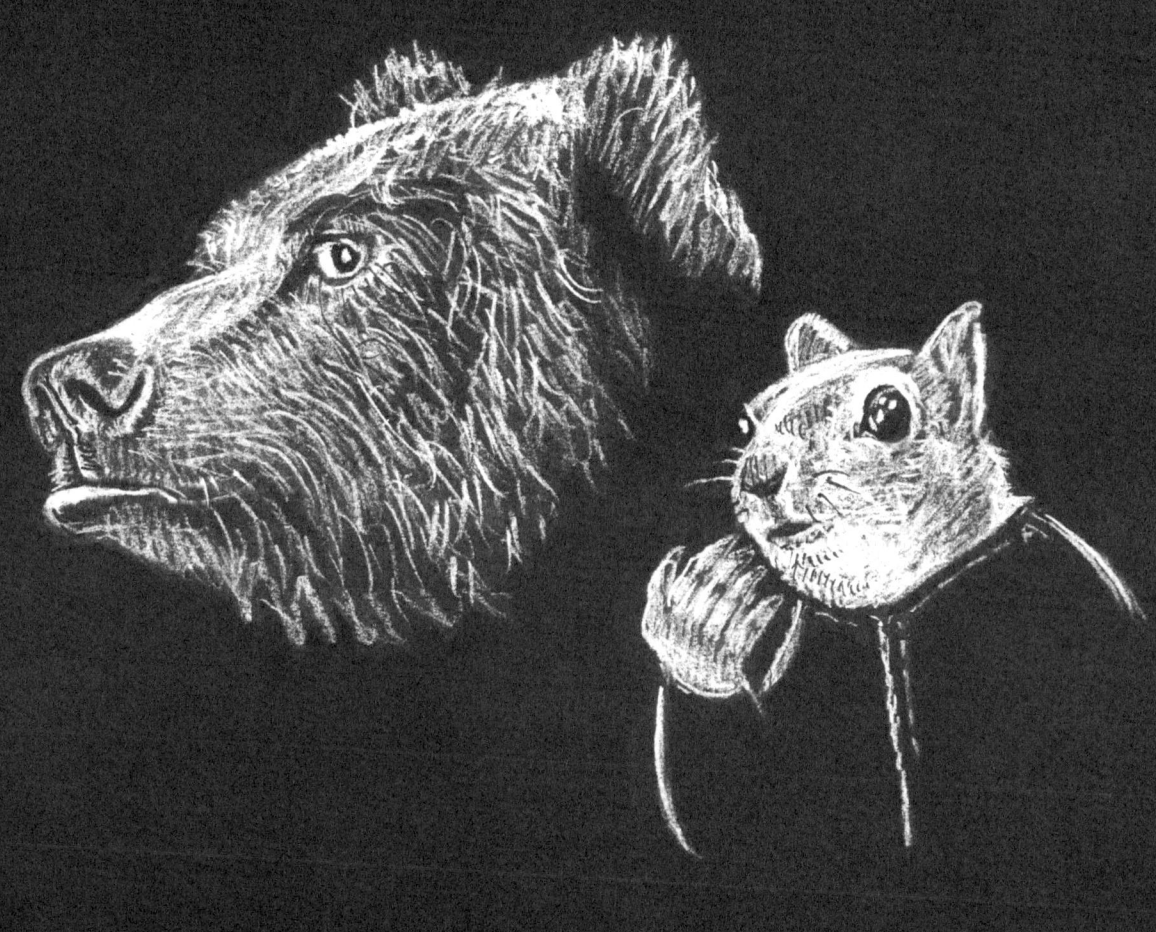

You're in a troubled relationship. You've tried to make it work, but your partner blames you, bullies, is unreasonably jealous or controlling.

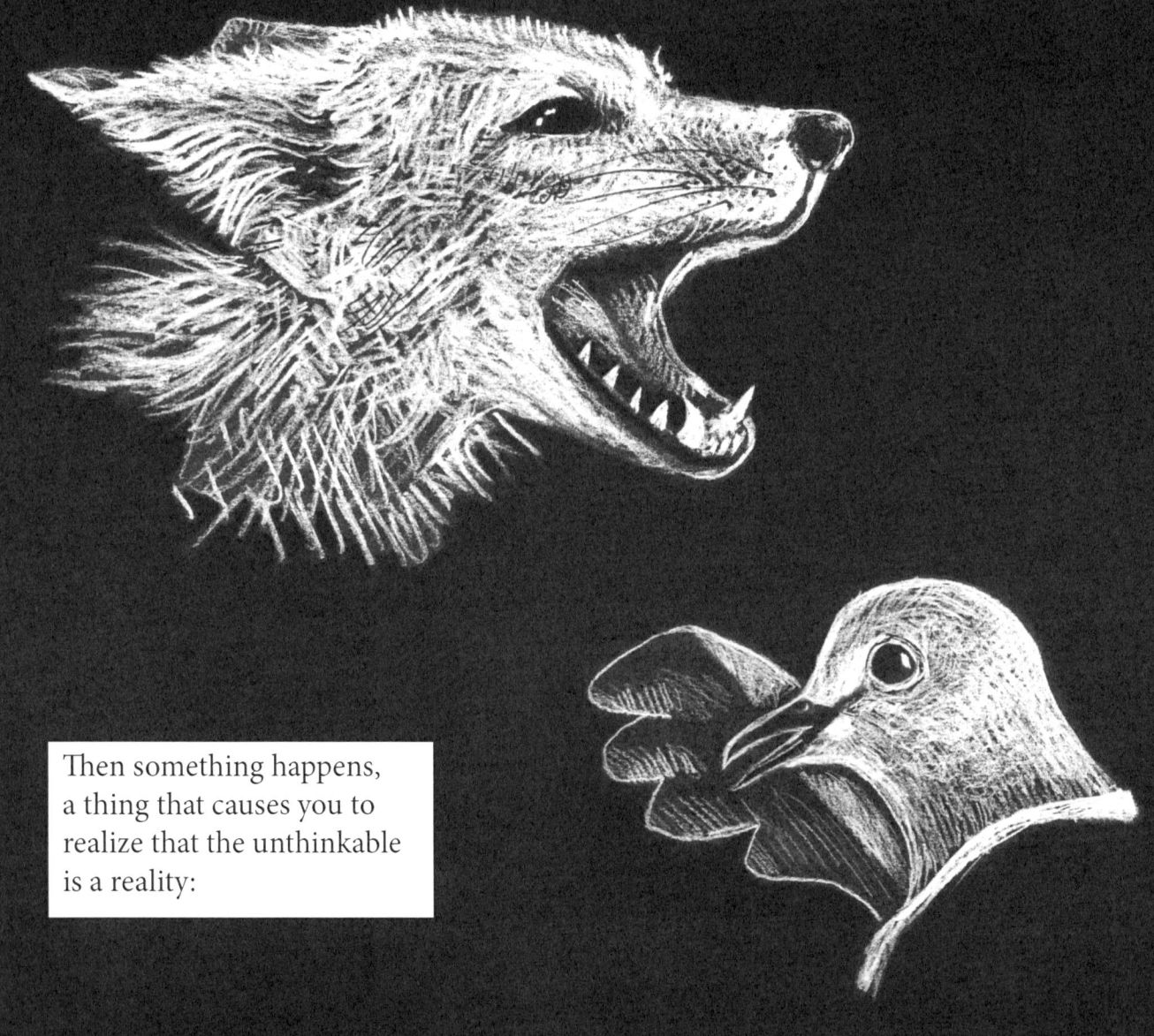

Then something happens, a thing that causes you to realize that the unthinkable is a reality:

I'm in an abusive relationship. I'm in danger.

I HAVE TO ESCAPE, BUT IT WON'T BE EASY. MANY NEVER DO.

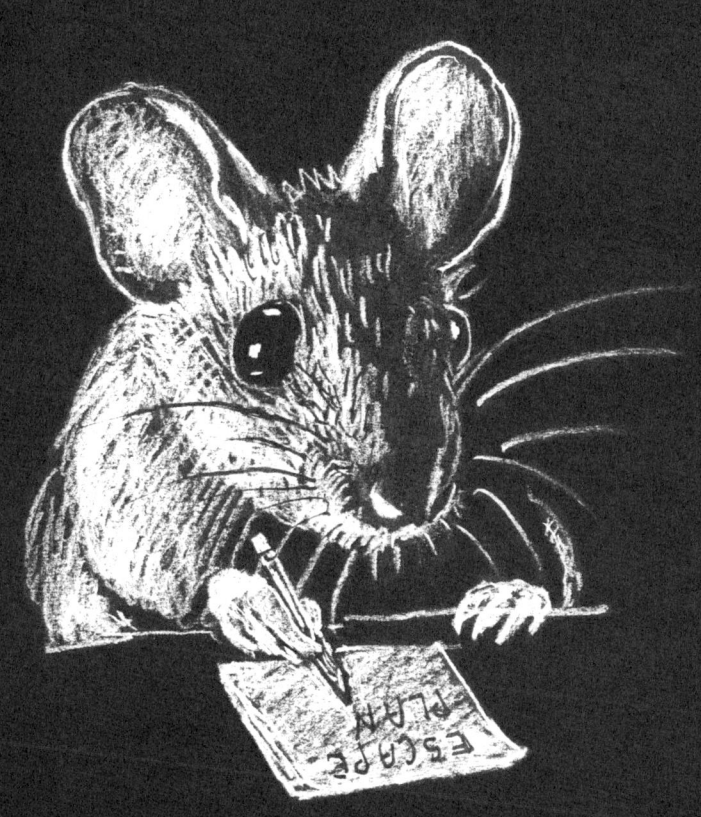

85% OF DOMESTIC VIOLENCE ATTACKS ARE ON WOMEN

15% OF WOMEN AND 4% OF MEN IN THE US HAVE BEEN INJURED AS A RESULT OF PHYSICAL VIOLENCE BY AN INTIMATE PARTNER

1527 WOMEN AND 510 MEN WERE KILLED BY AN INTIMATE PARTNER IN THE US IN 2017

HALF OF ALL MURDERS OF WOMEN ARE COMMITTED BY A FORMER OR CURRENT ROMANTIC PARTNER

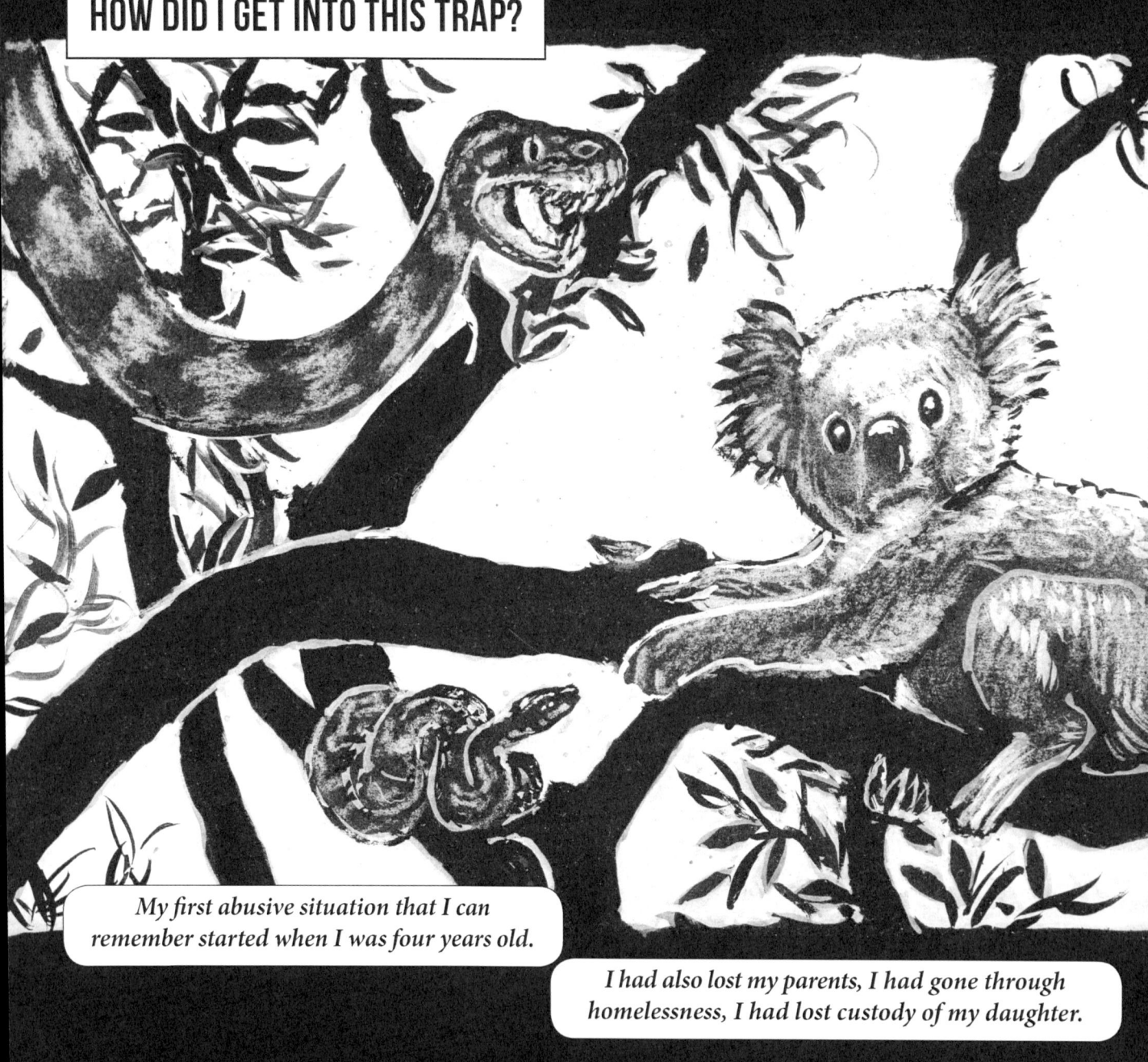

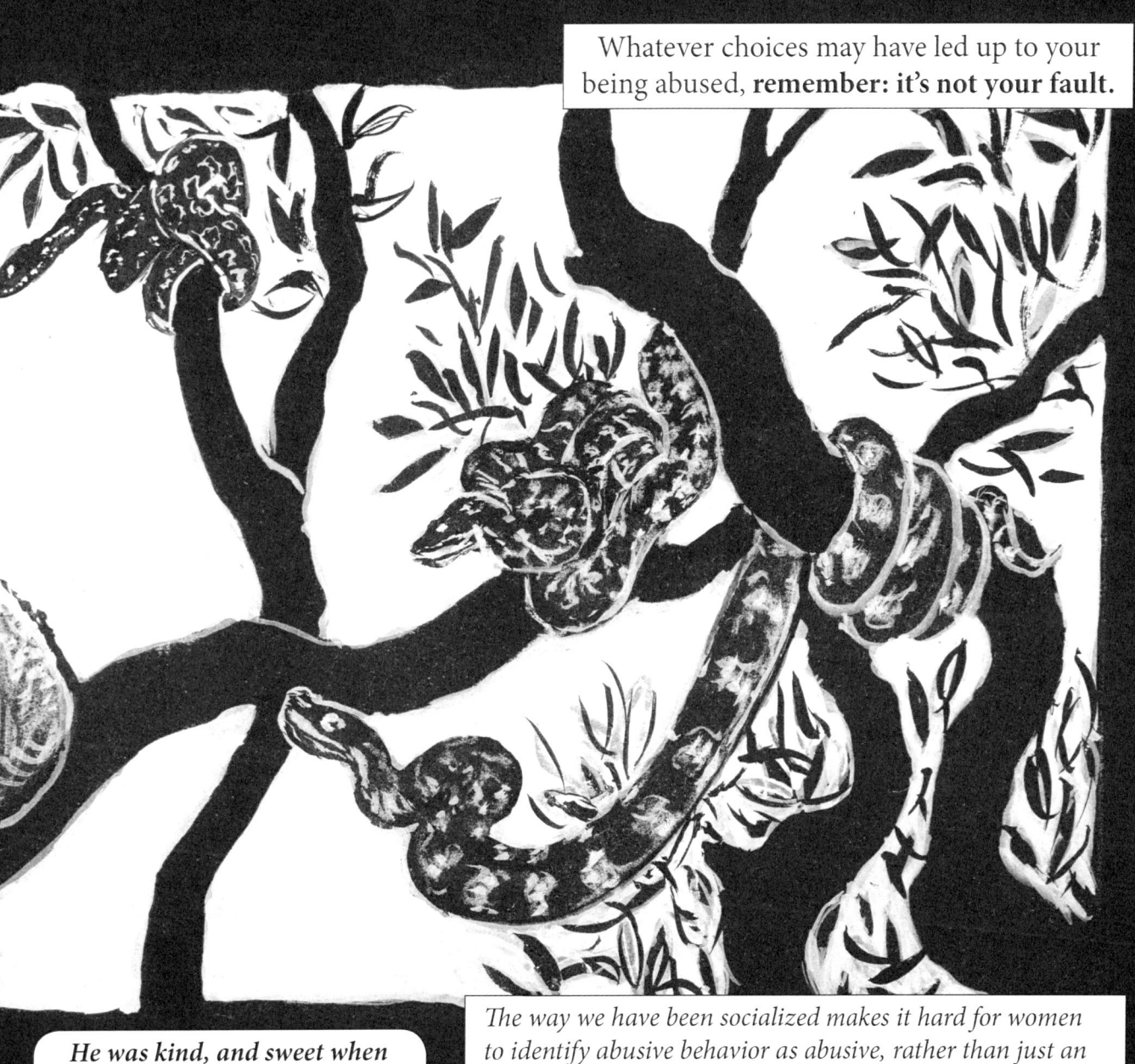

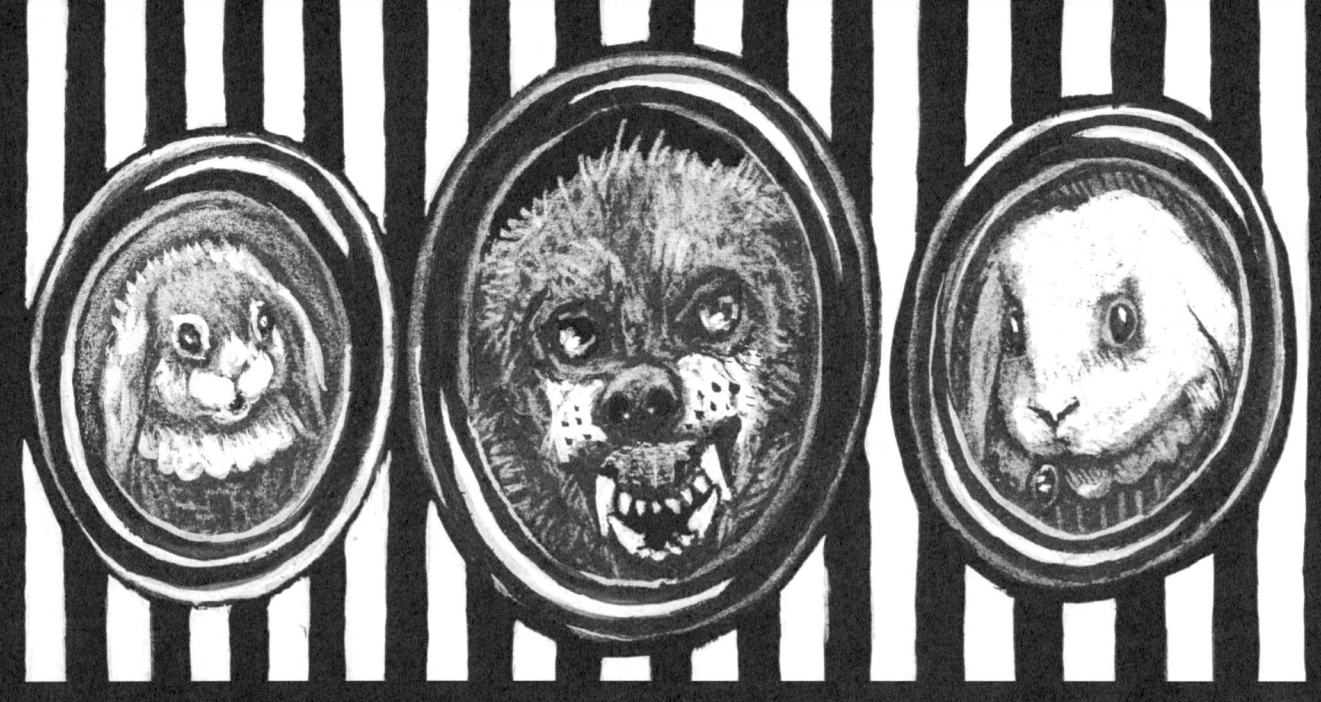

My early family life taught me to accept the unacceptable and inappropriate.

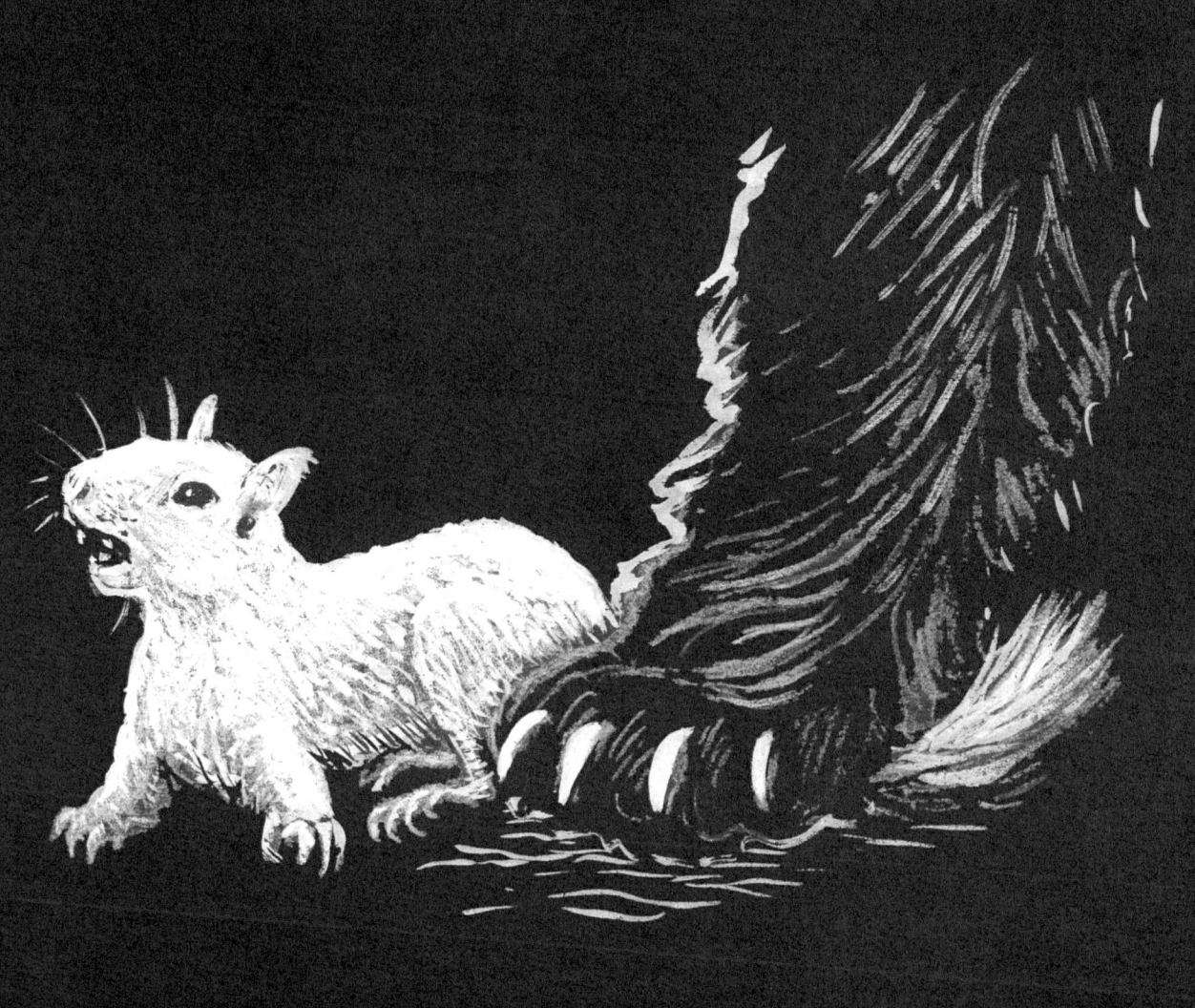

The only relationship advice I got from my Mom was that a boy shows his affection through name calling and hitting.

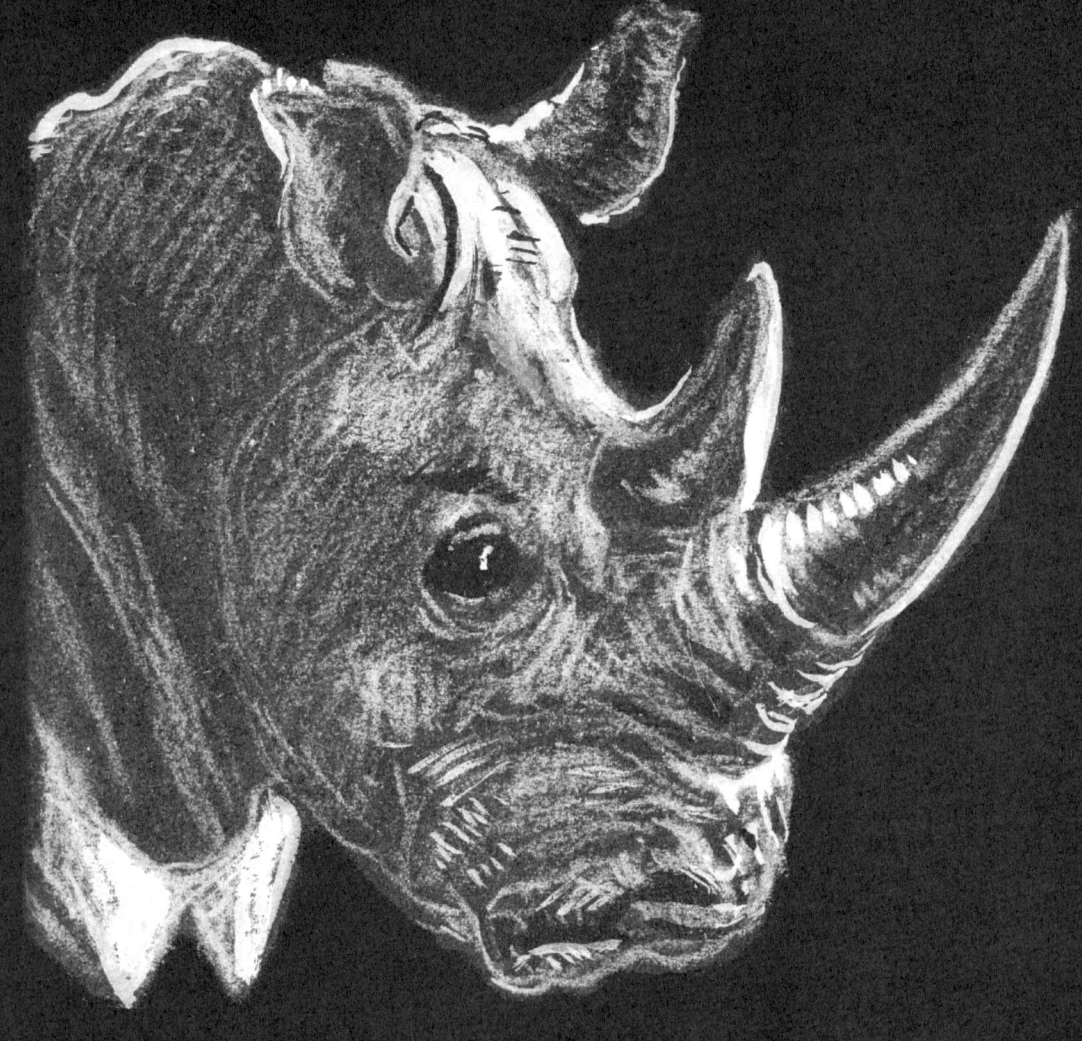

Narcissists target challenges – people who they perceive to be better than them – to latch on to and bring down.

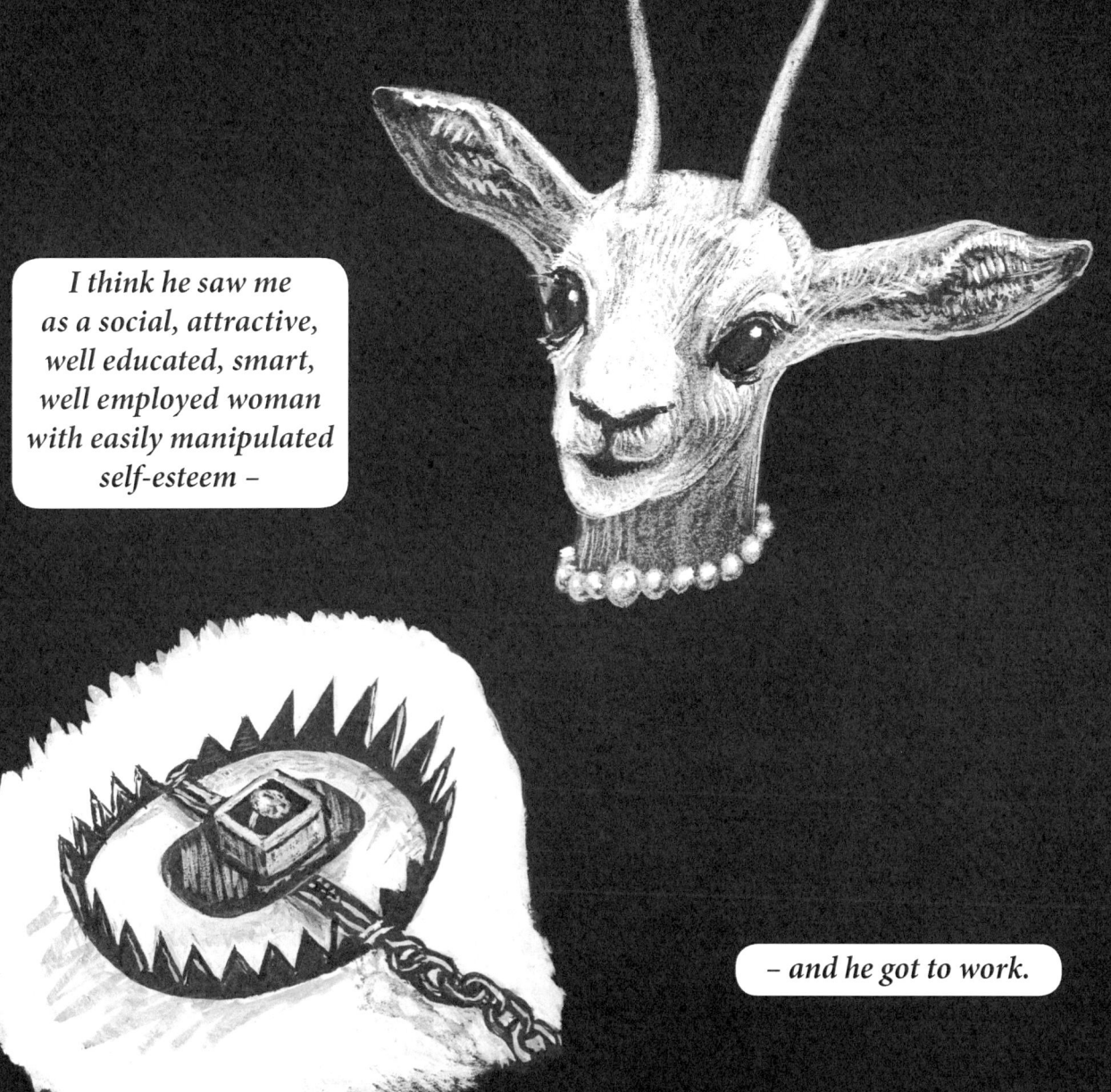

I KNEW I WAS IN AN ABUSIVE RELATIONSHIP WHEN...

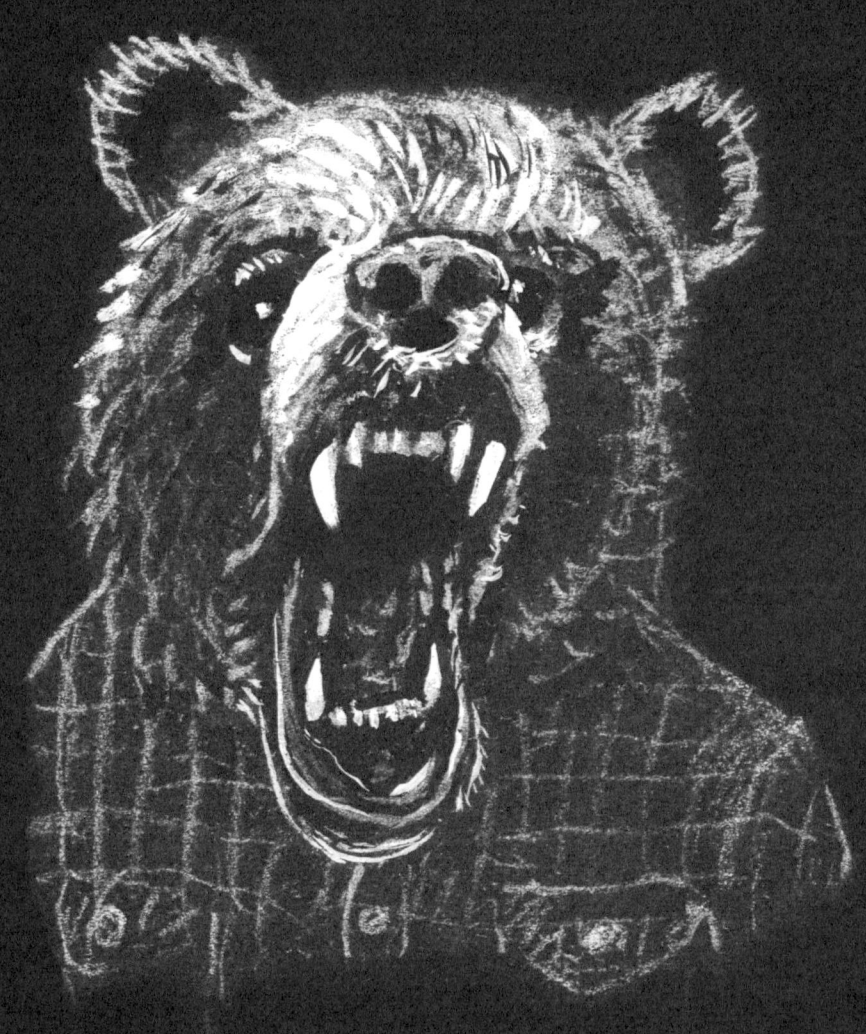

...He called me all sorts of names.

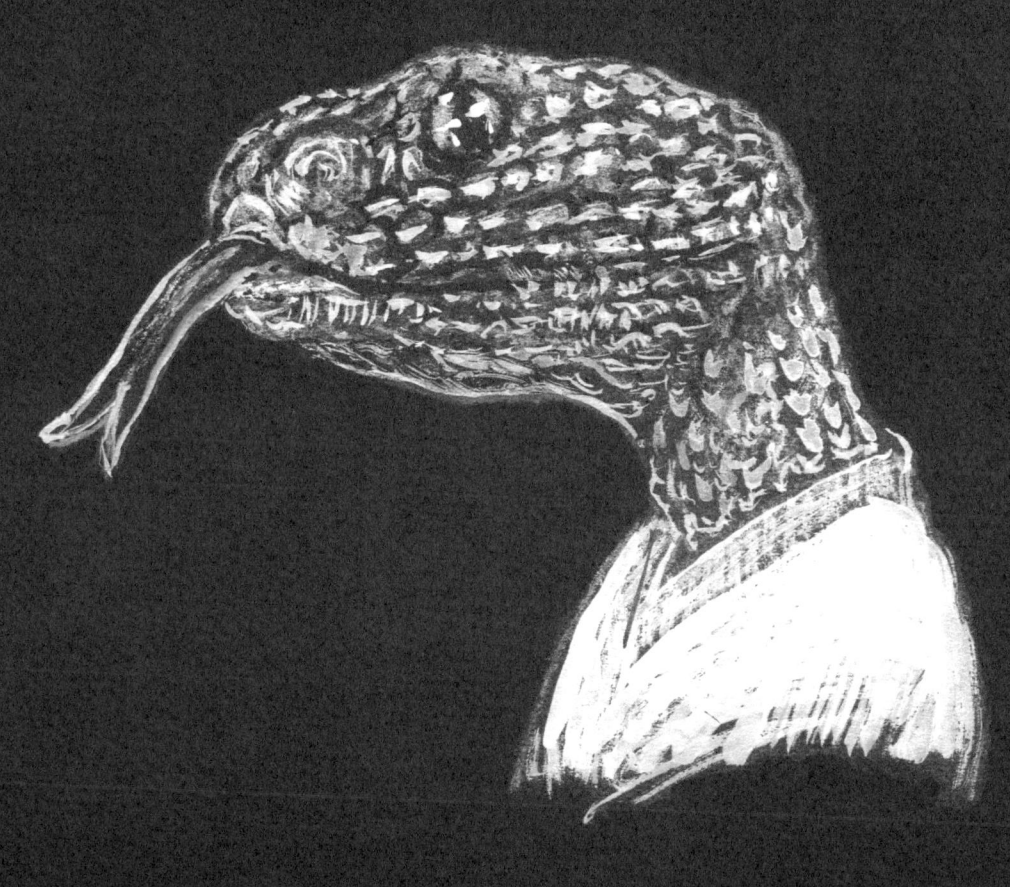

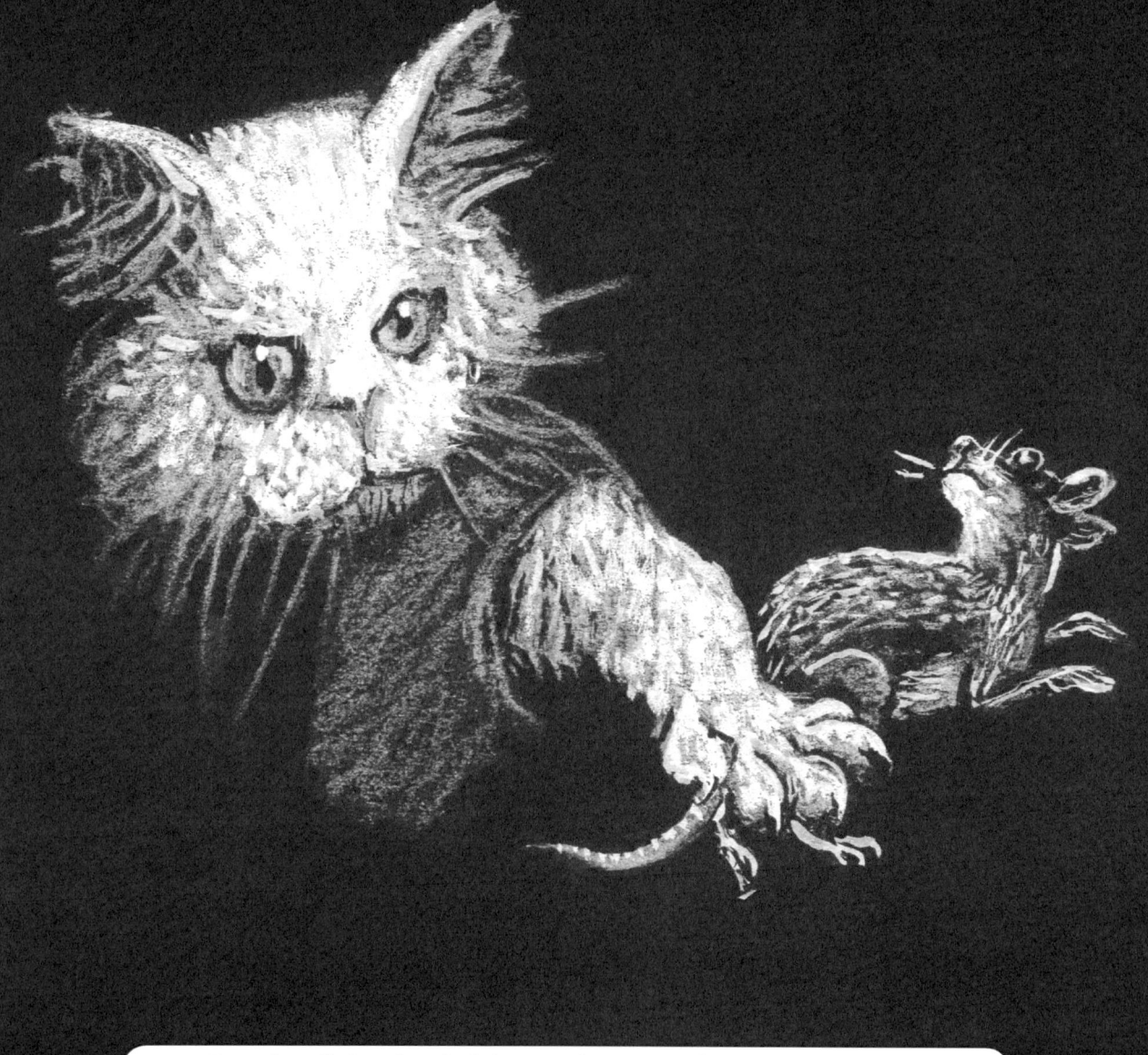

...I realized that he didn't care how comfortable I was. Ever.

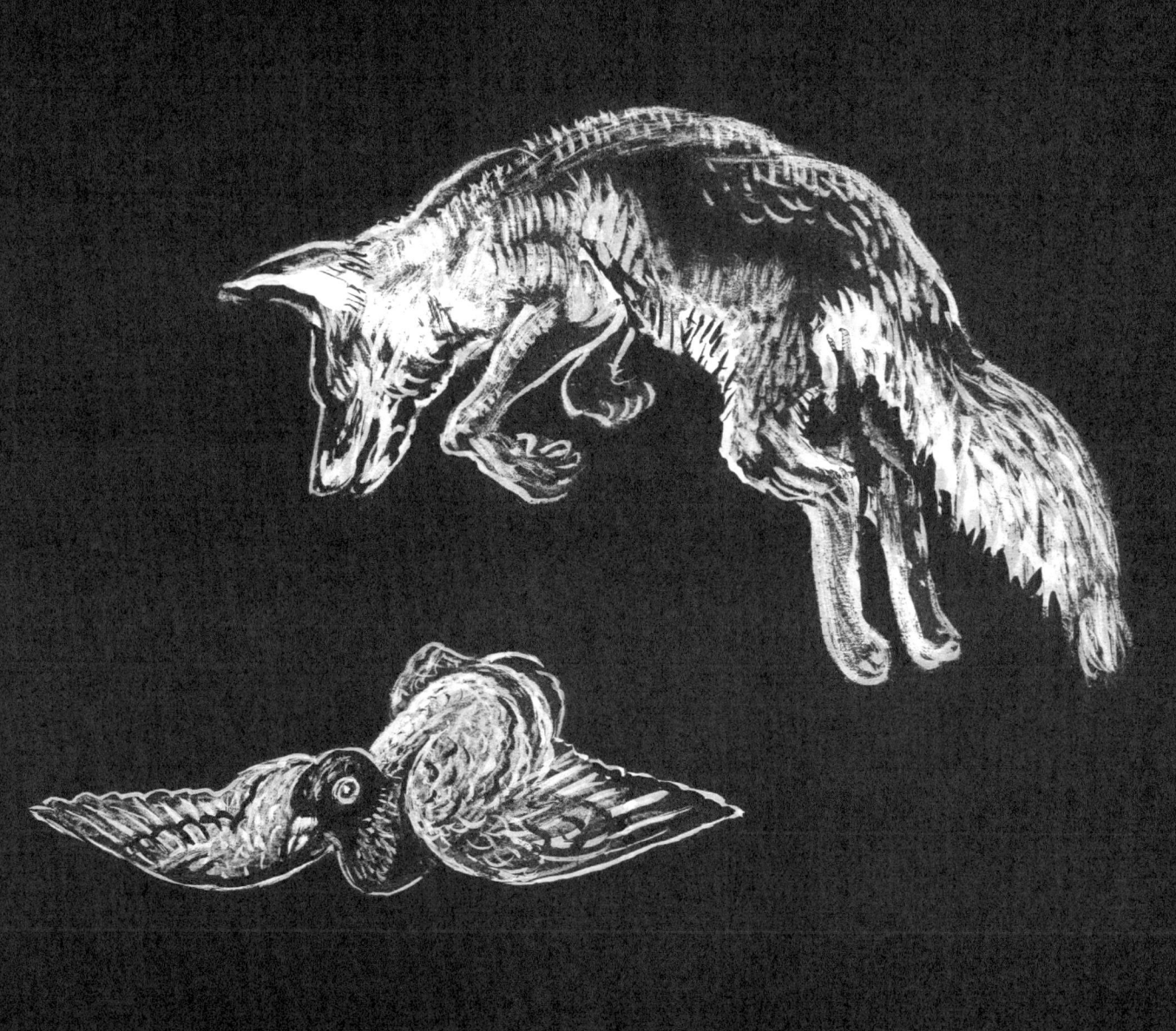

...He threw me down on the ground and kicked me.

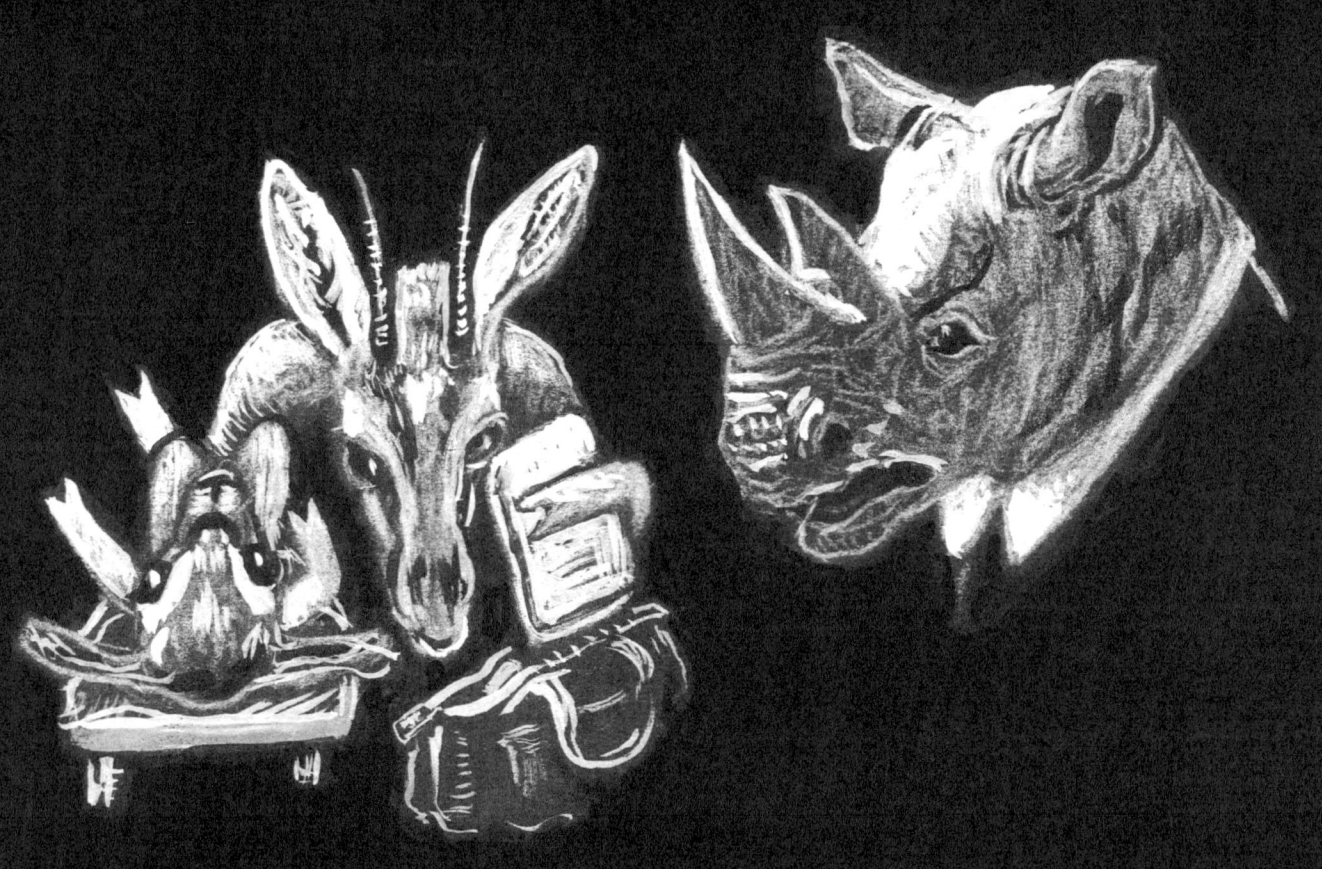

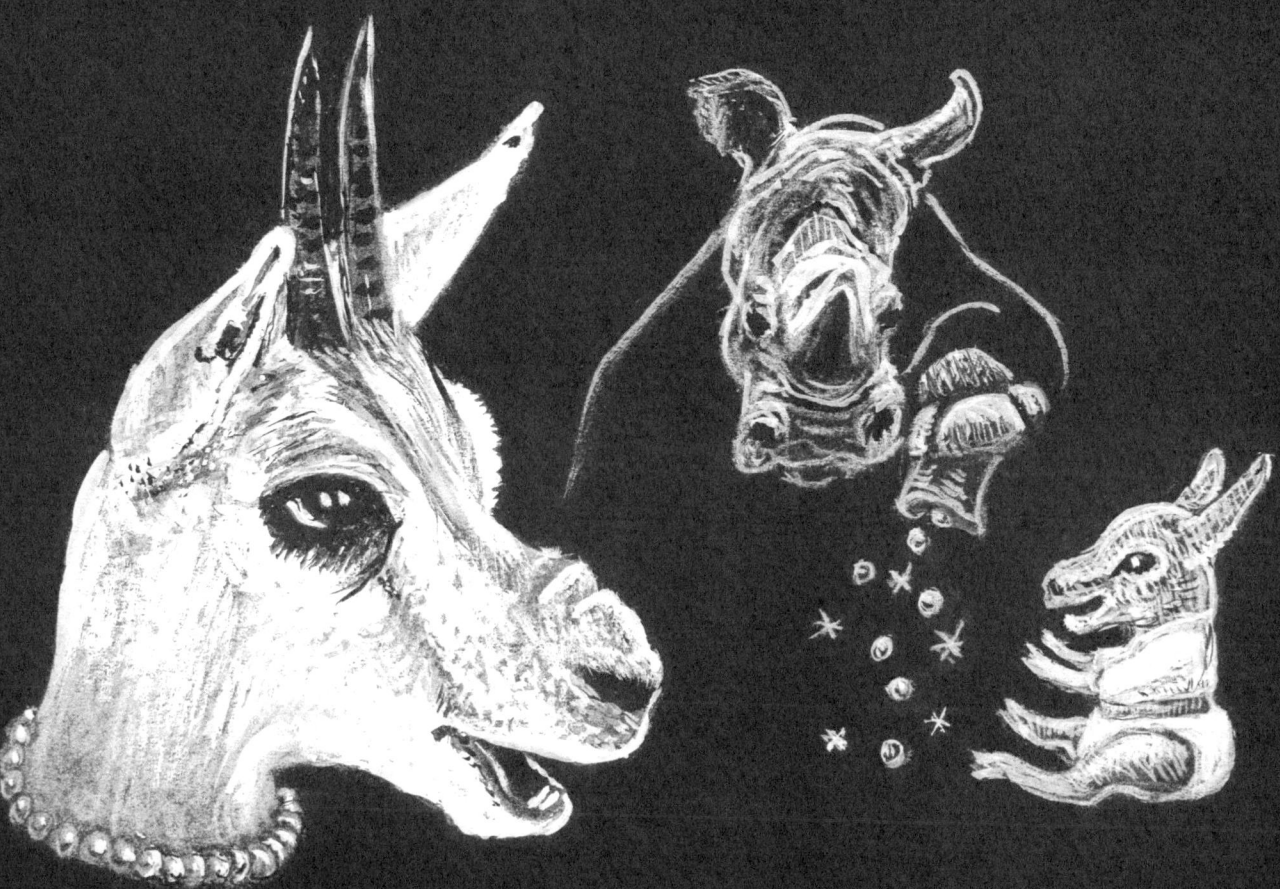

WHAT'S STOPPING ME FROM GETTING AWAY?

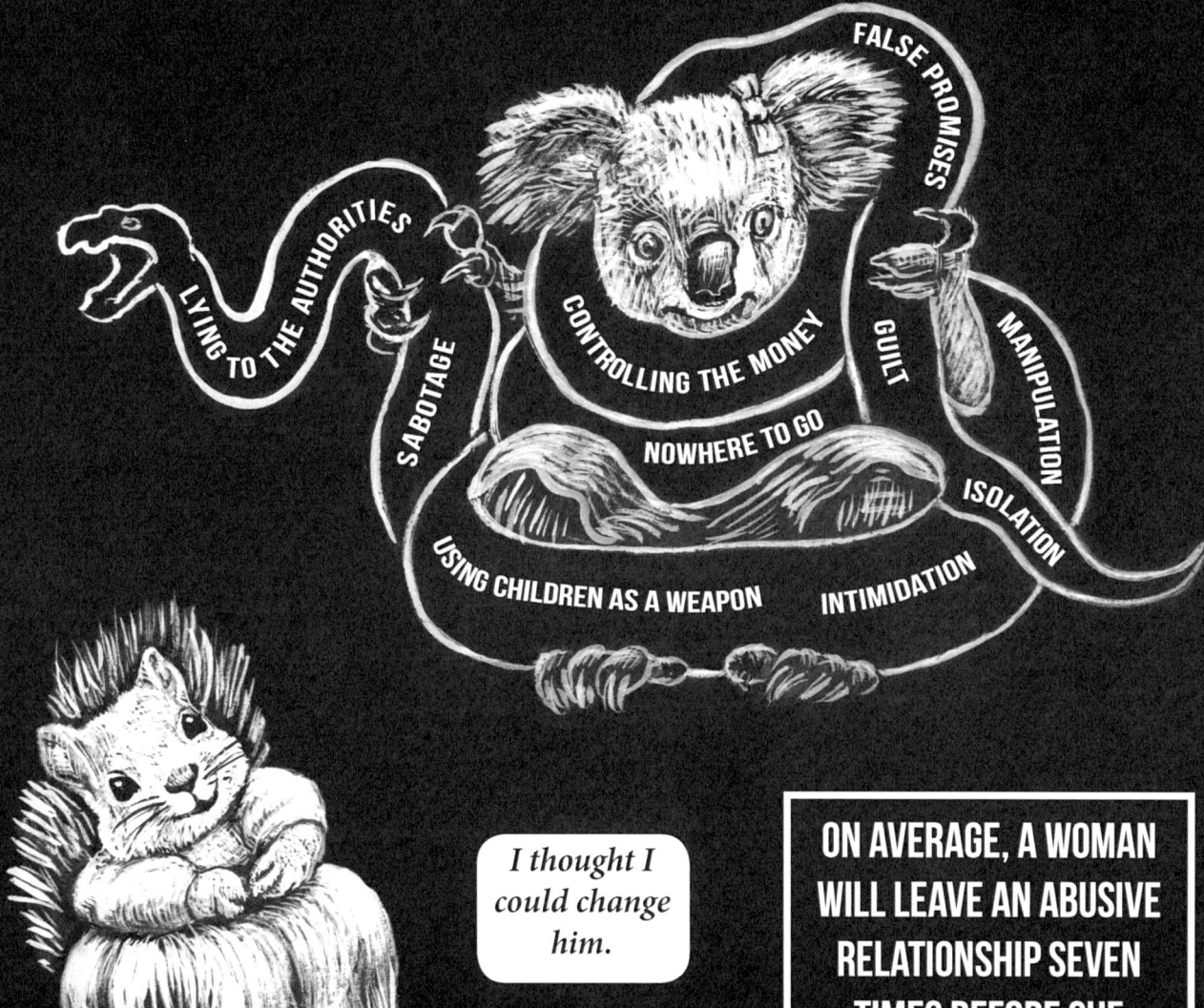

FALSE PROMISES · LYING TO THE AUTHORITIES · SABOTAGE · CONTROLLING THE MONEY · GUILT · MANIPULATION · NOWHERE TO GO · ISOLATION · USING CHILDREN AS A WEAPON · INTIMIDATION

I thought I could change him.

ON AVERAGE, A WOMAN WILL LEAVE AN ABUSIVE RELATIONSHIP SEVEN TIMES BEFORE SHE LEAVES FOR GOOD

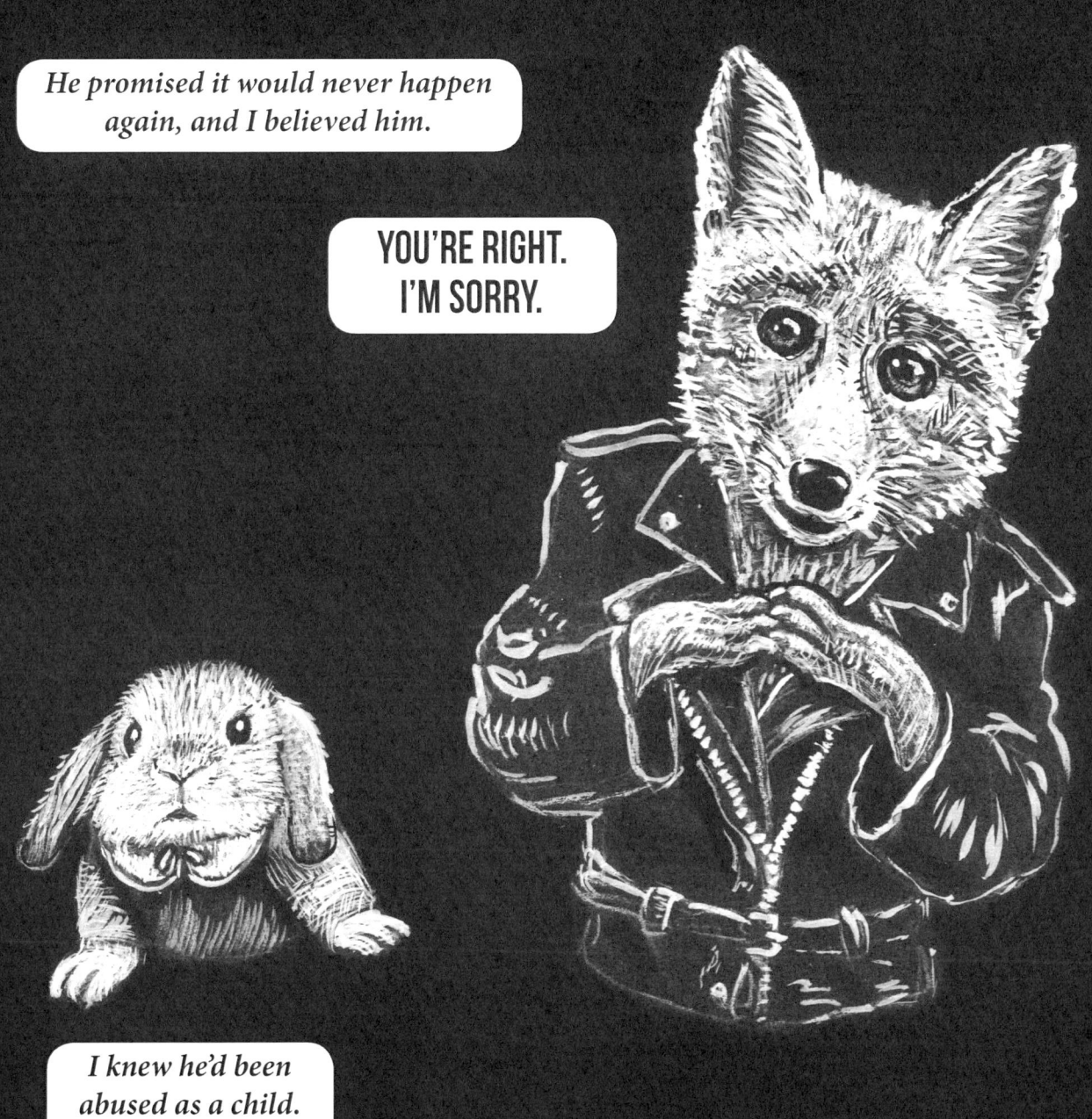

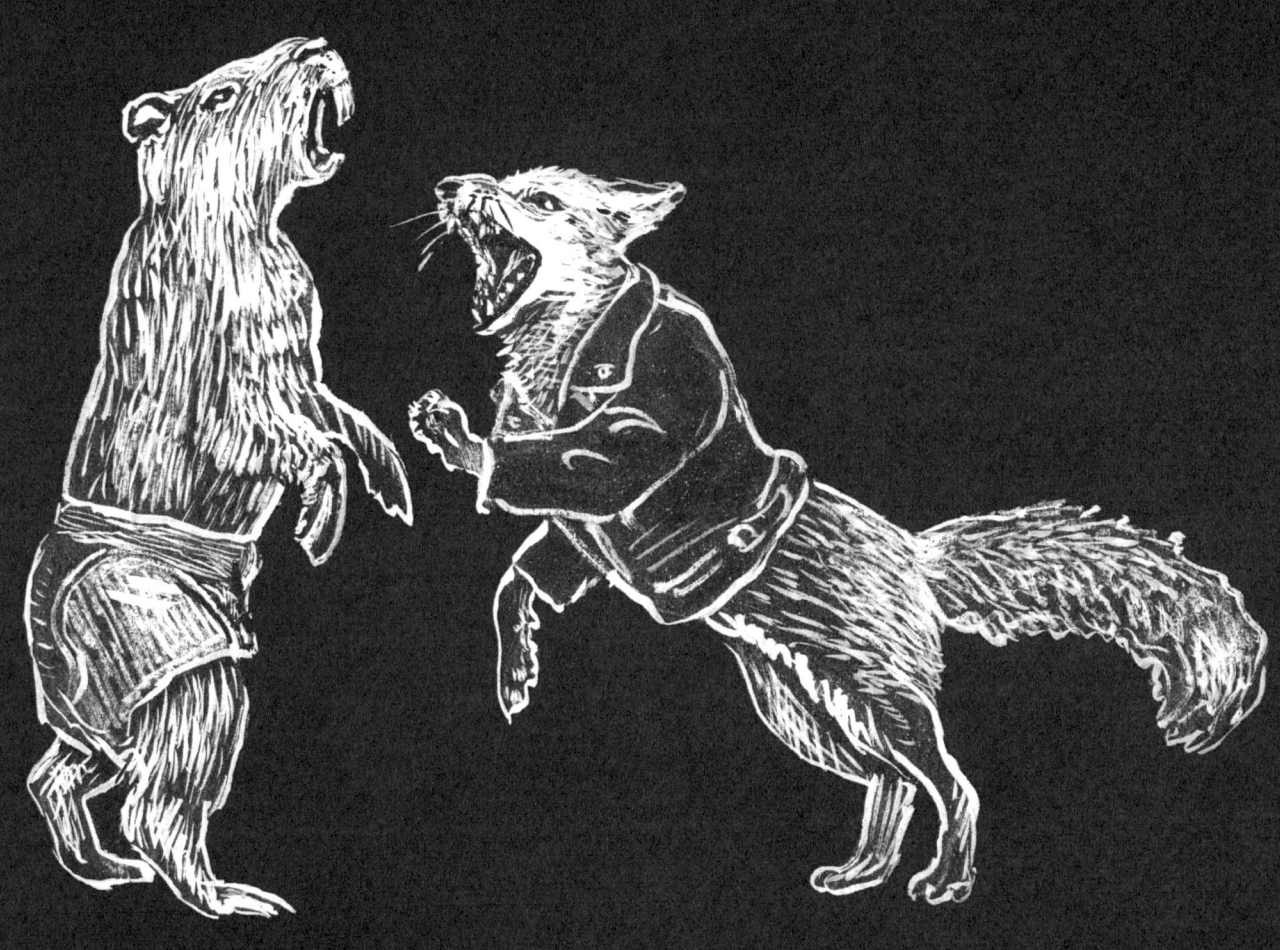

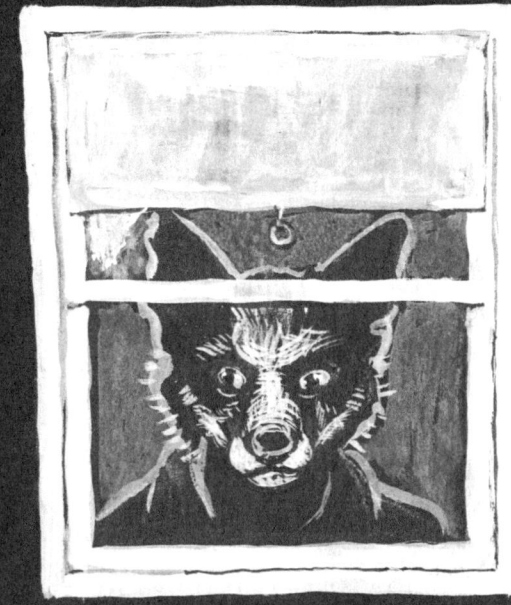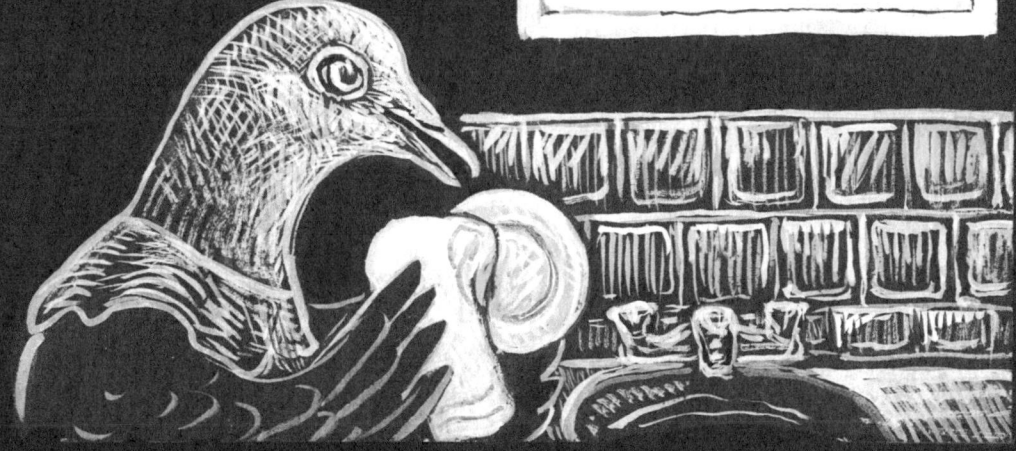

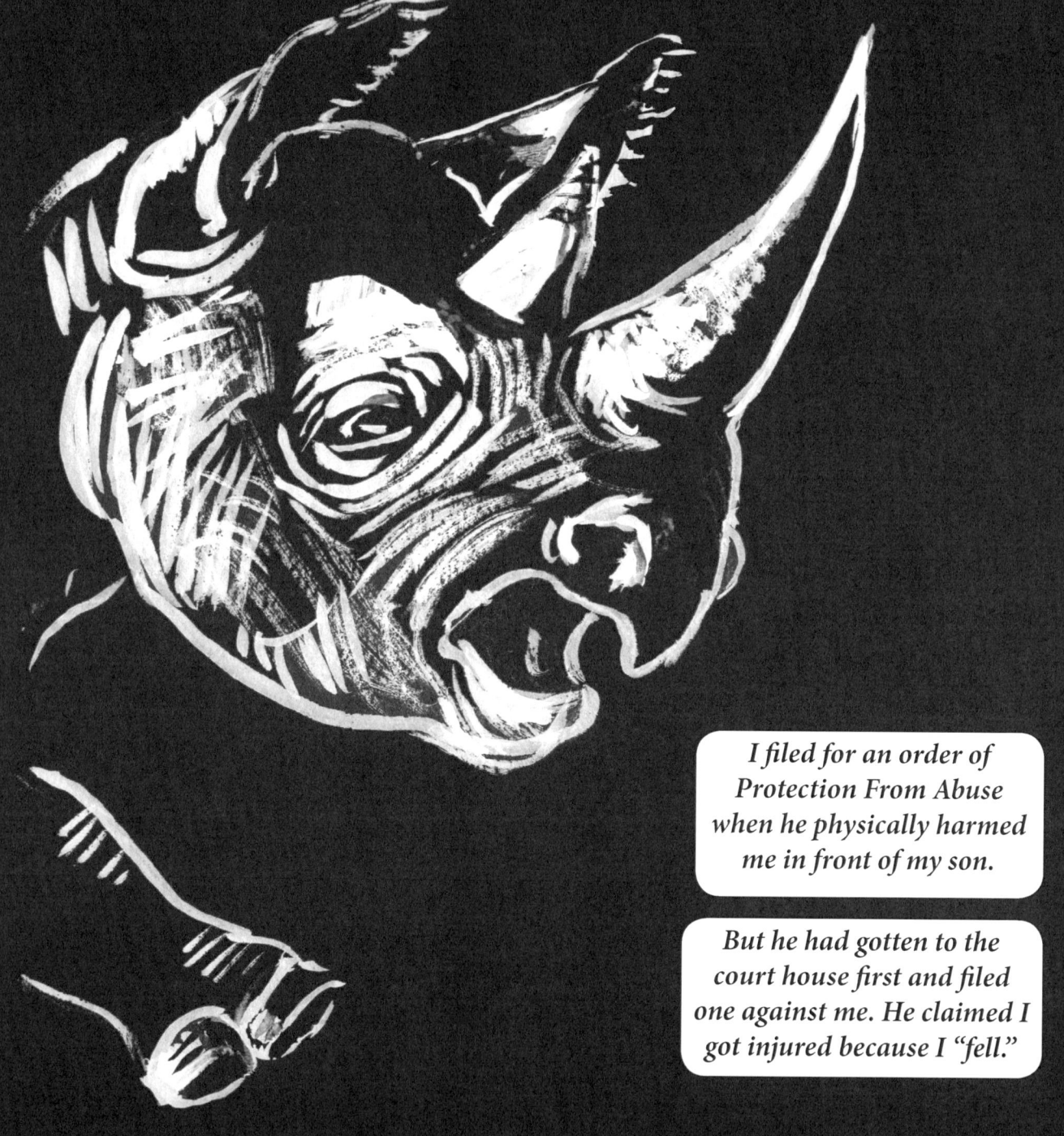

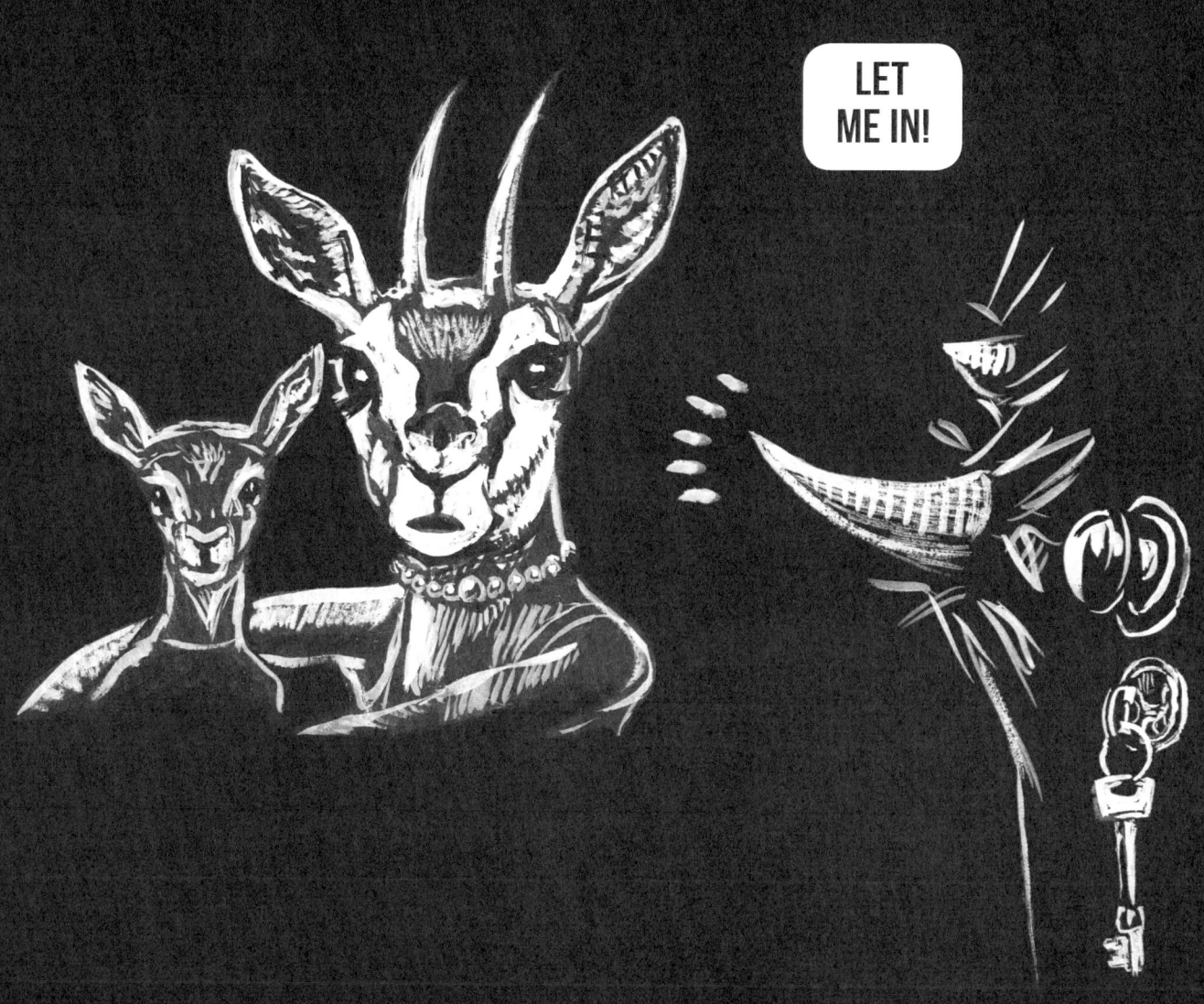

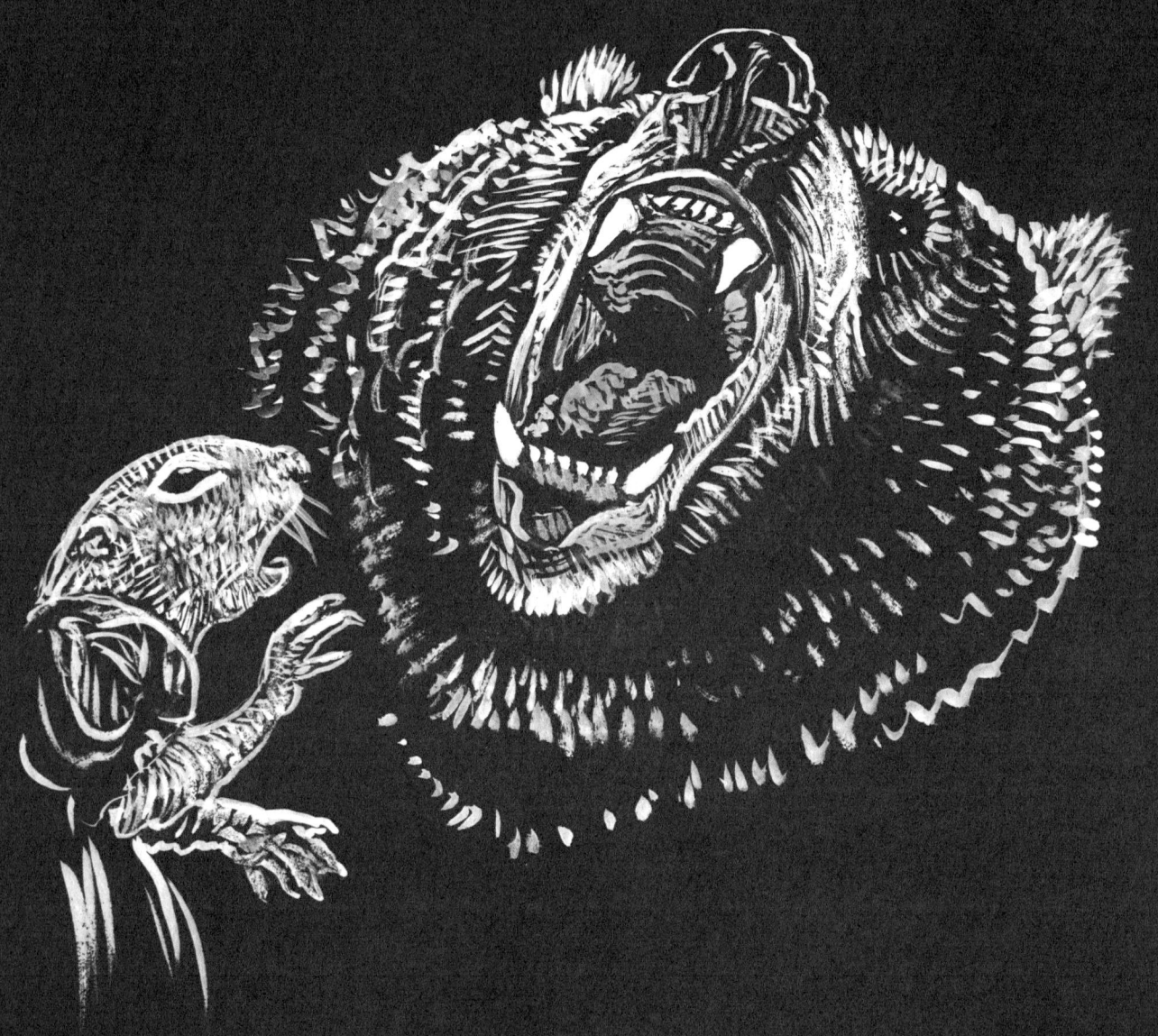

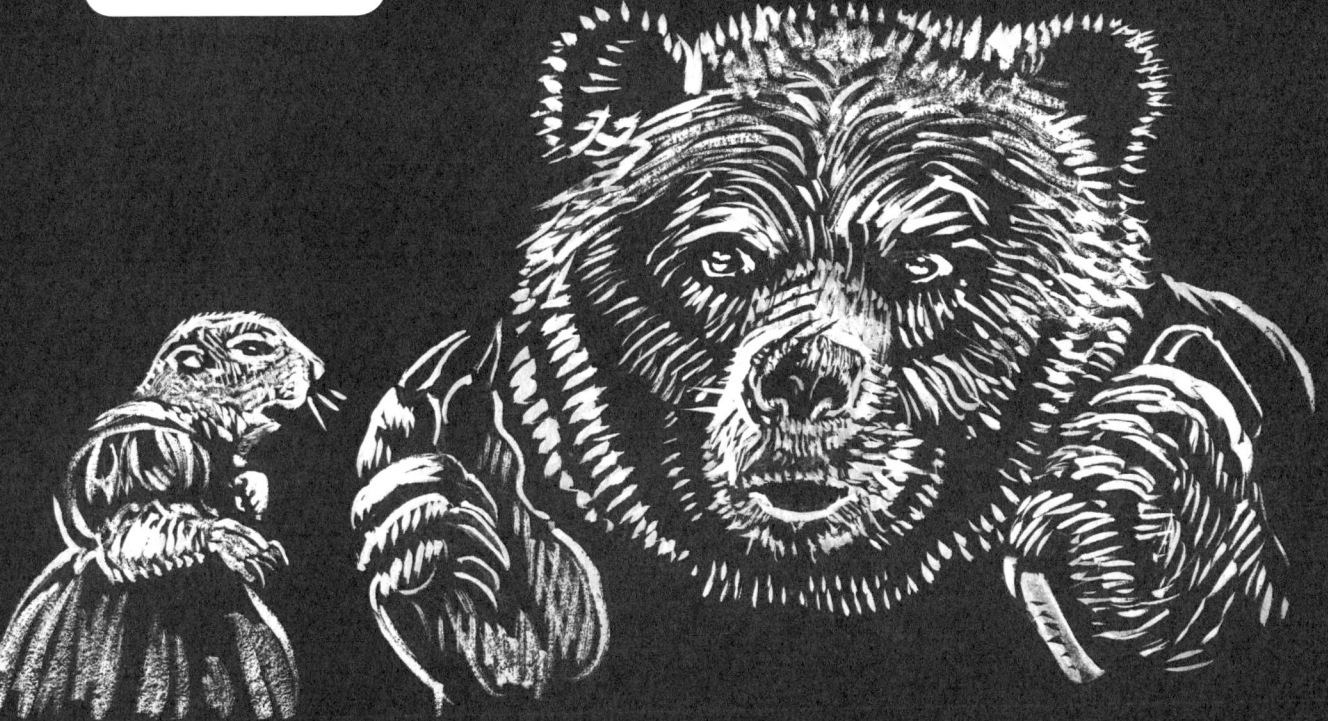

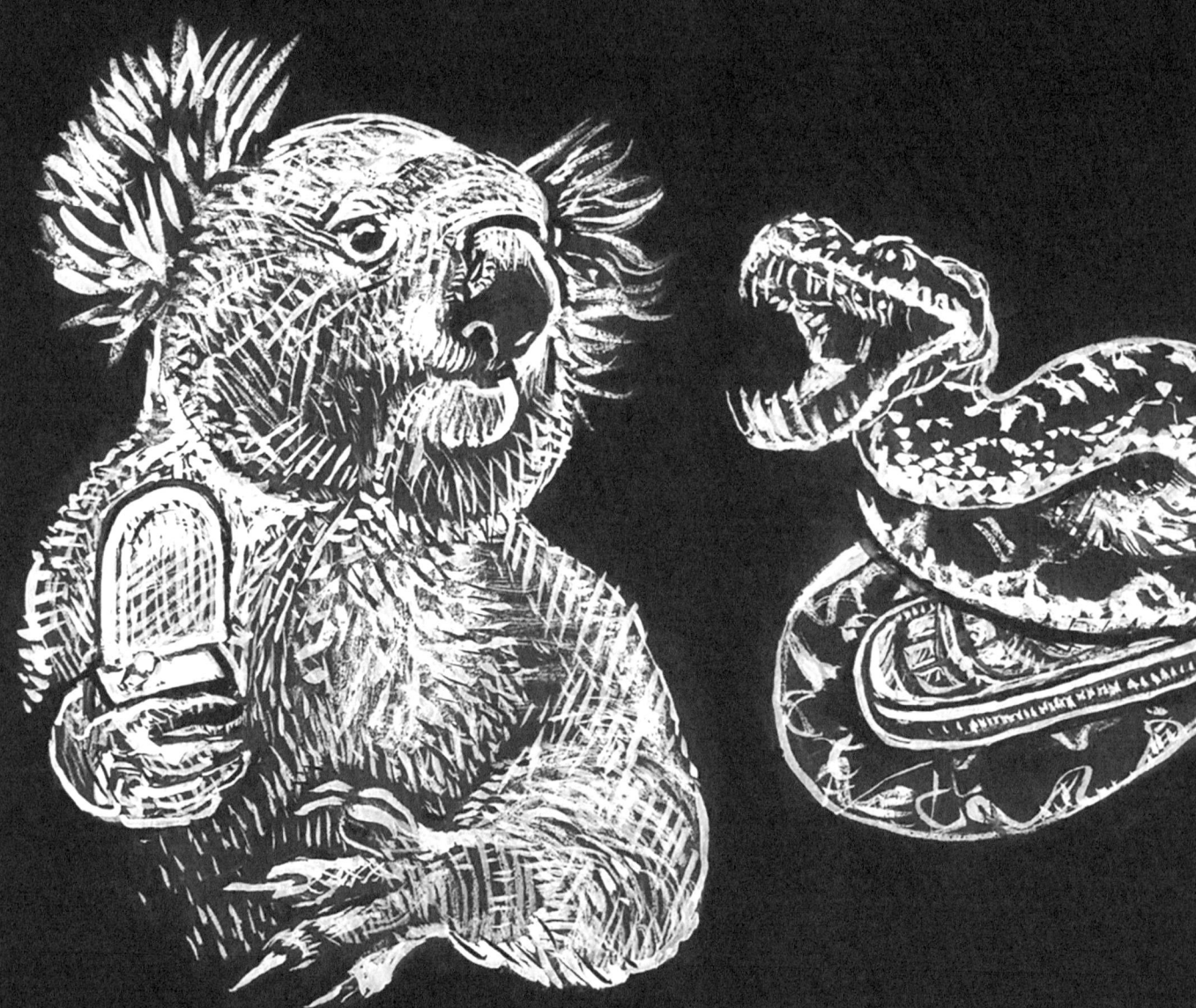

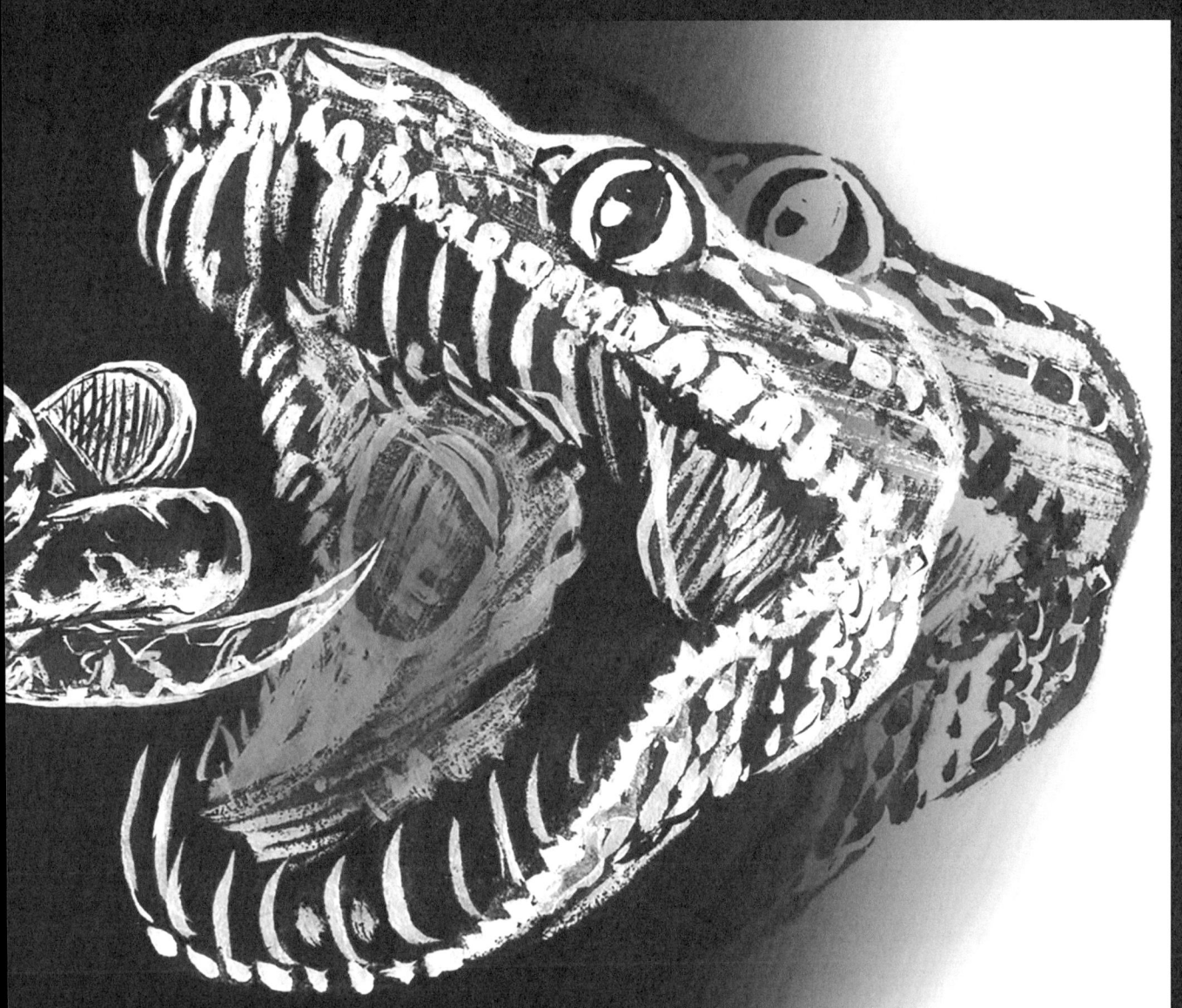

Things got very bad very quickly at that point.

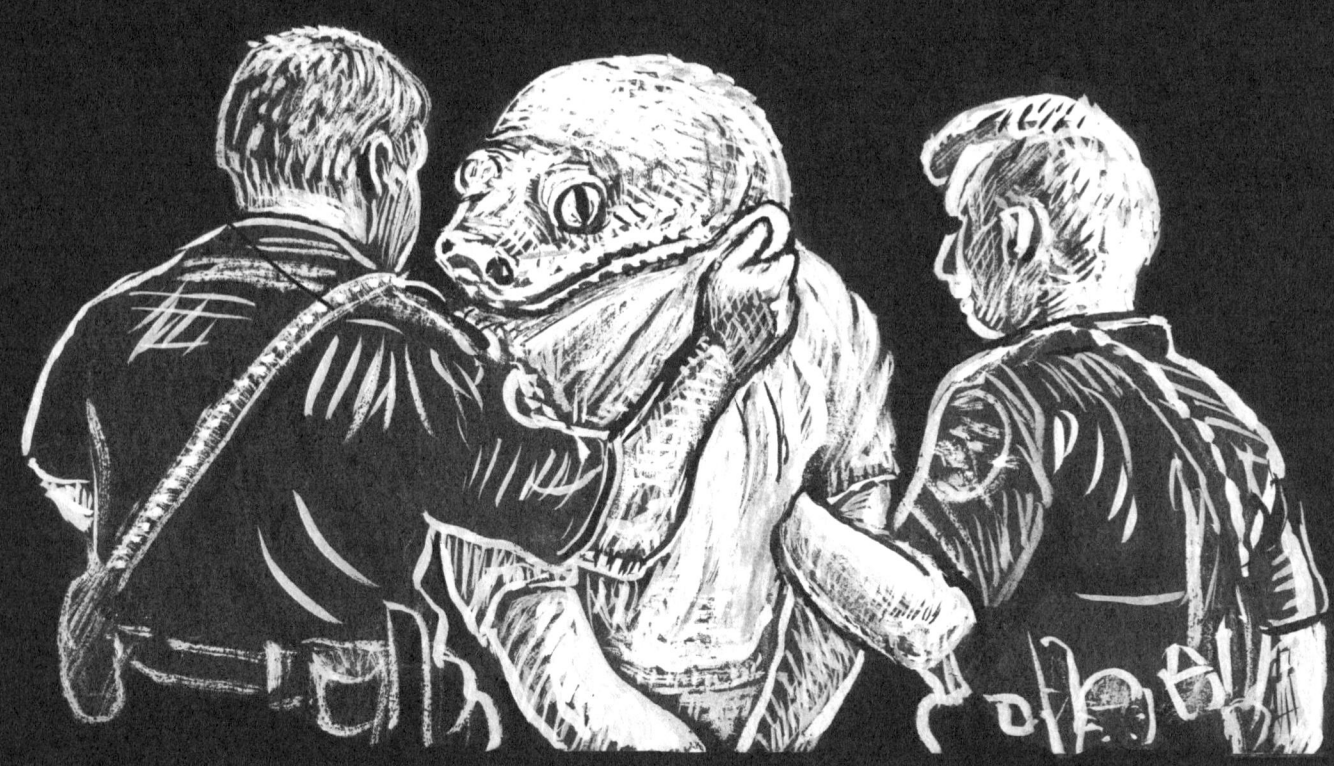

I CAN'T EVEN IMAGINE LEAVING.

It's not uncommon for a battered woman not to fully comprehend that she is experiencing abuse.

This is because when a person experiences severe trauma, their mind goes into denial. This detachment allows them to function and survive. But the traumatized person tends to see each incident as an isolated event, not as part of a pattern of abuse.

They may blame themselves, or make excuses for the abuser. They feel completely dependent. Between extremes of hurt and being comforted, they experience "traumatic bonding."

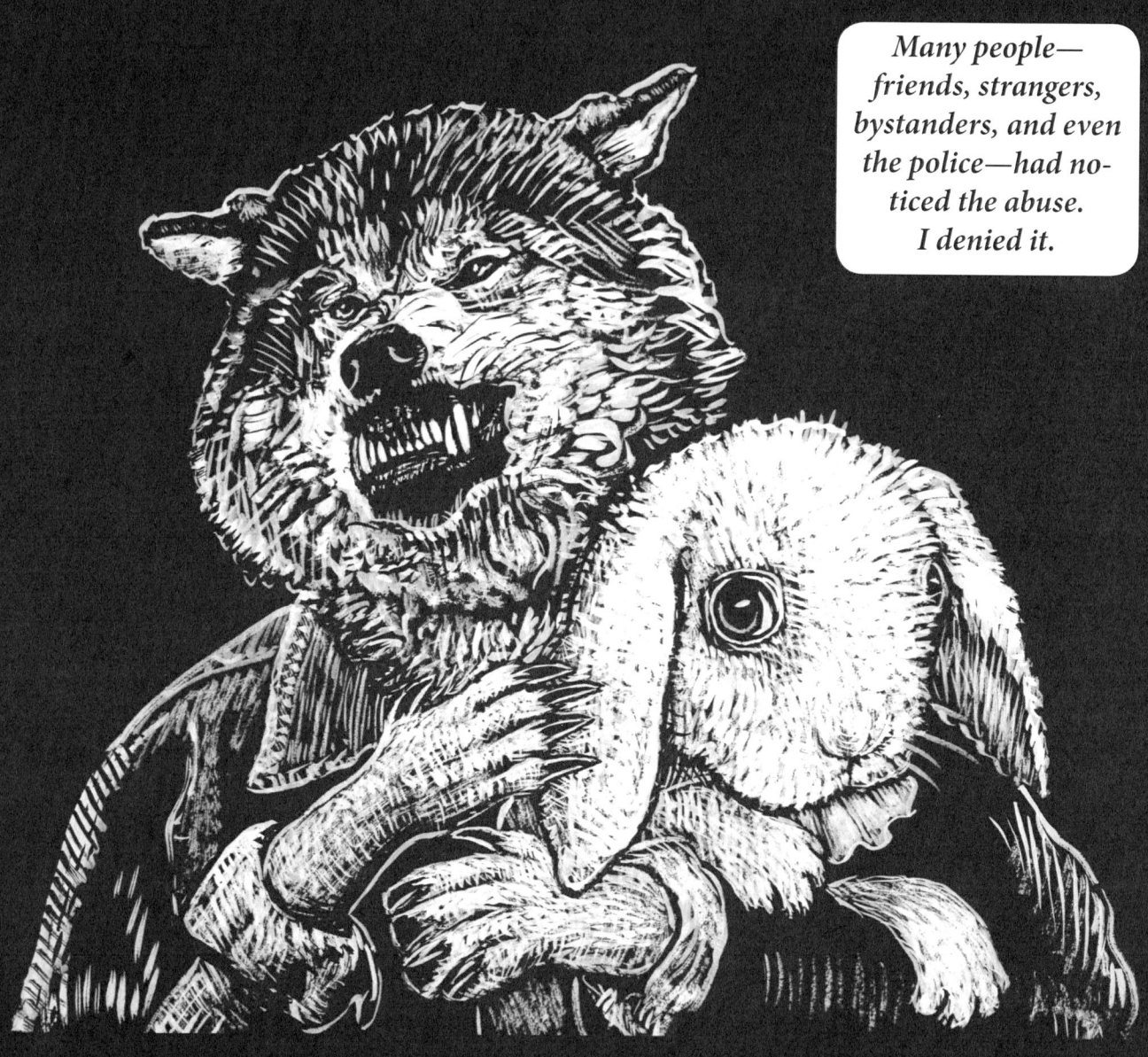

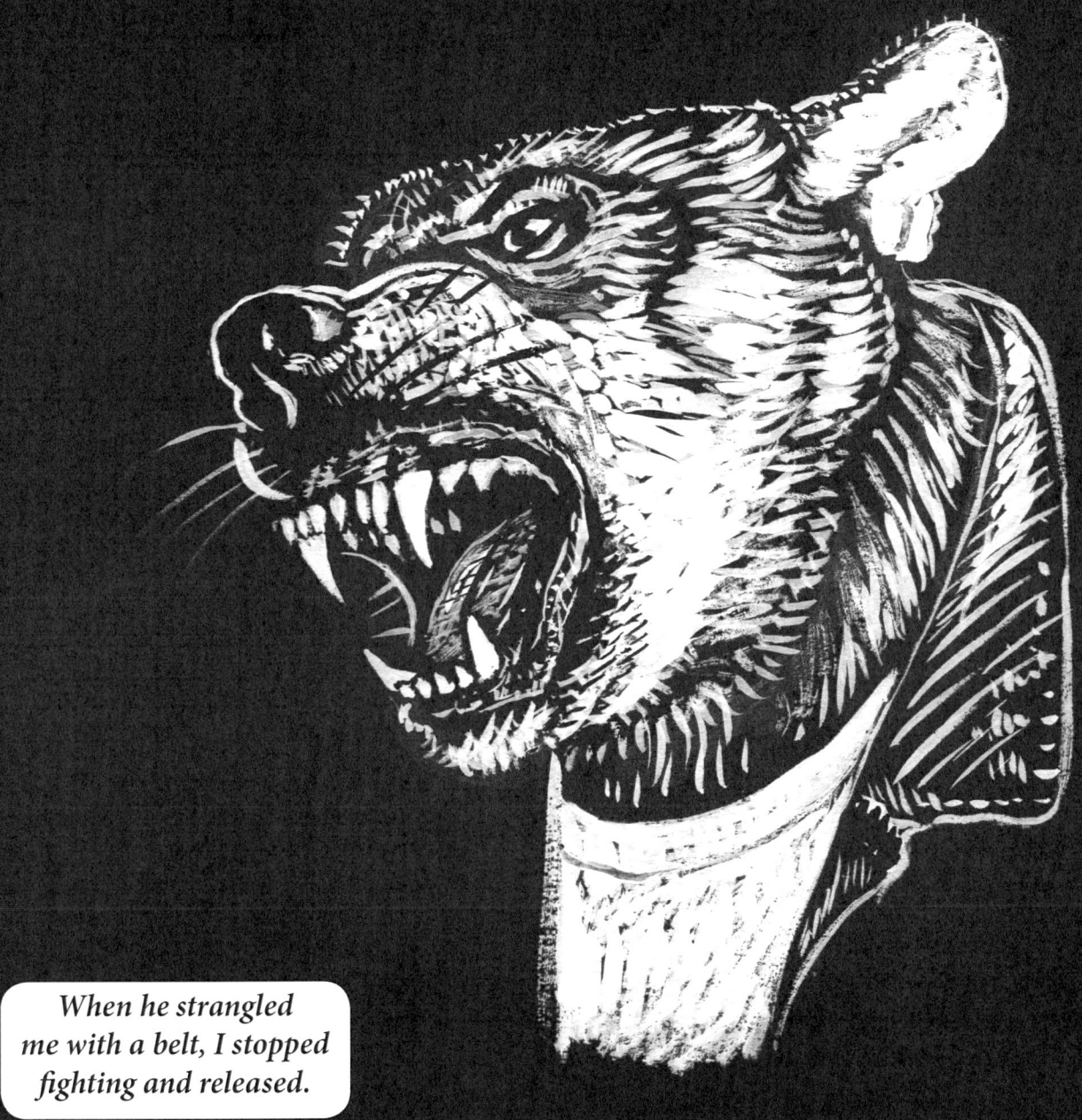

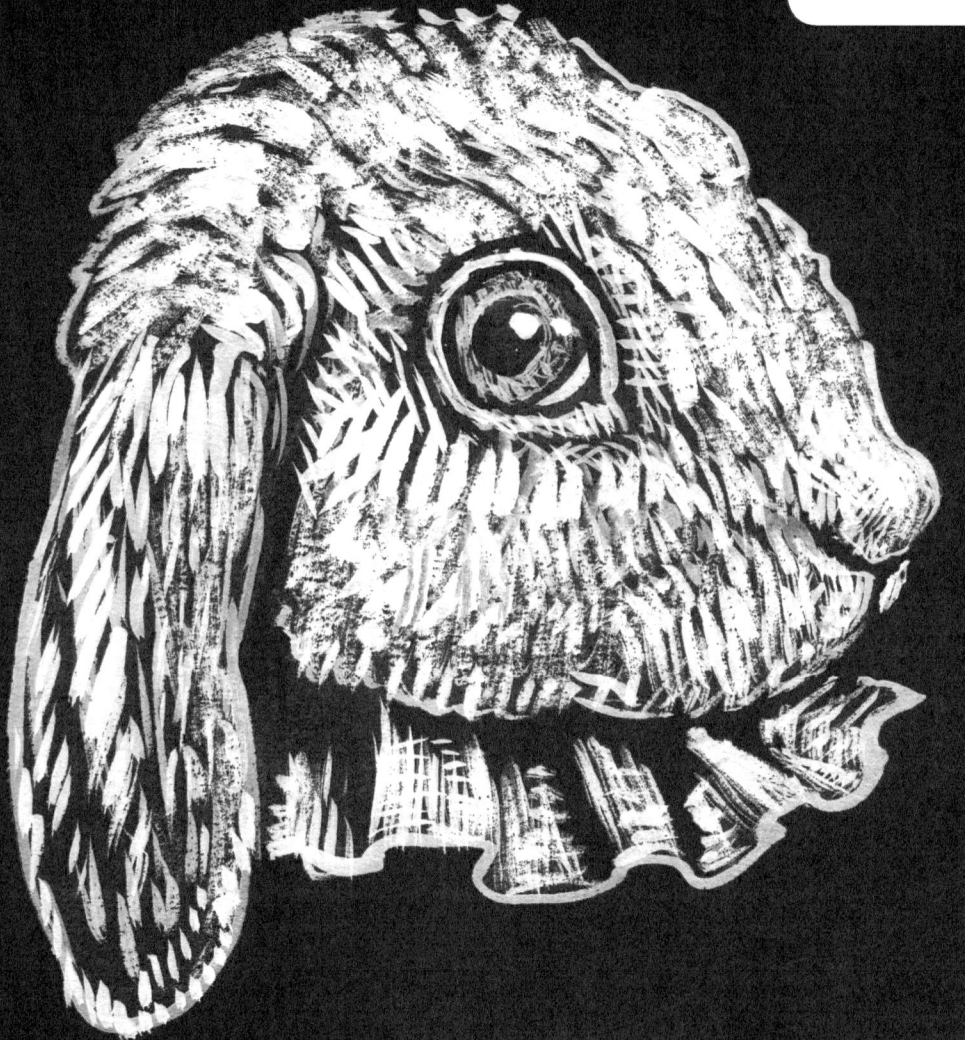

...When I looked into the mirror, I was stunned.

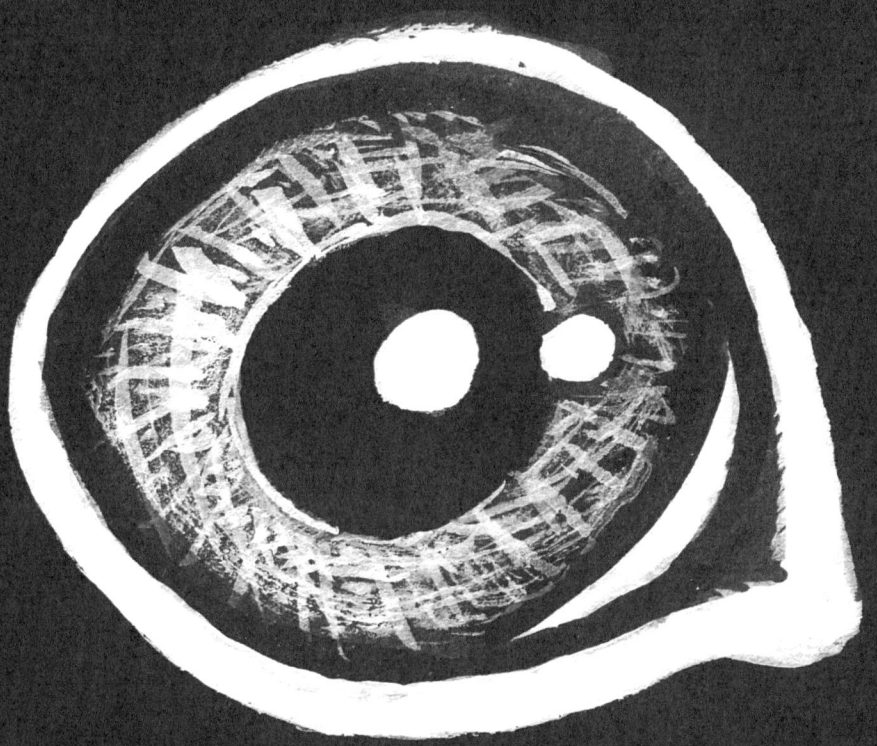

My nose was fractured, my eyes were bulging, my neck was covered in bruises, and there were shapes drawn on my cheeks and forehead in blood.
It was then I understood.

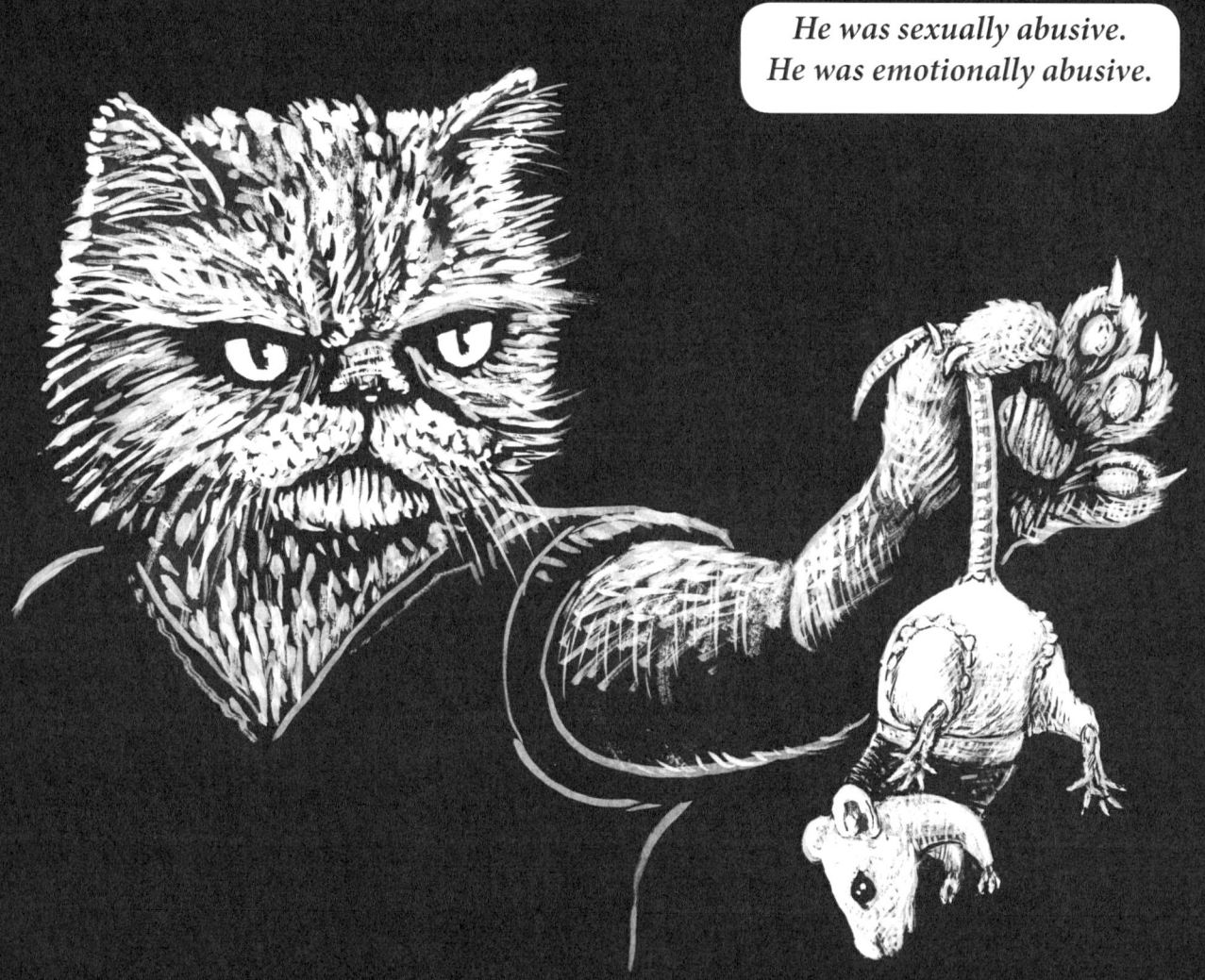

> NEARLY HALF OF ALL WOMEN IN ABUSIVE RELATIONSHIPS WILL ALSO BE SEXUALLY ASSAULTED DURING THE COURSE OF THE RELATIONSHIP

> SEXUAL VIOLENCE IN A RELATIONSHIP IS A FORM OF ASSAULT THAT CAUSES LASTING PHYSICAL AND PSYCHOLOGICAL DAMAGE

WHAT KIND OF INTERVENTION ISN'T HELPING?

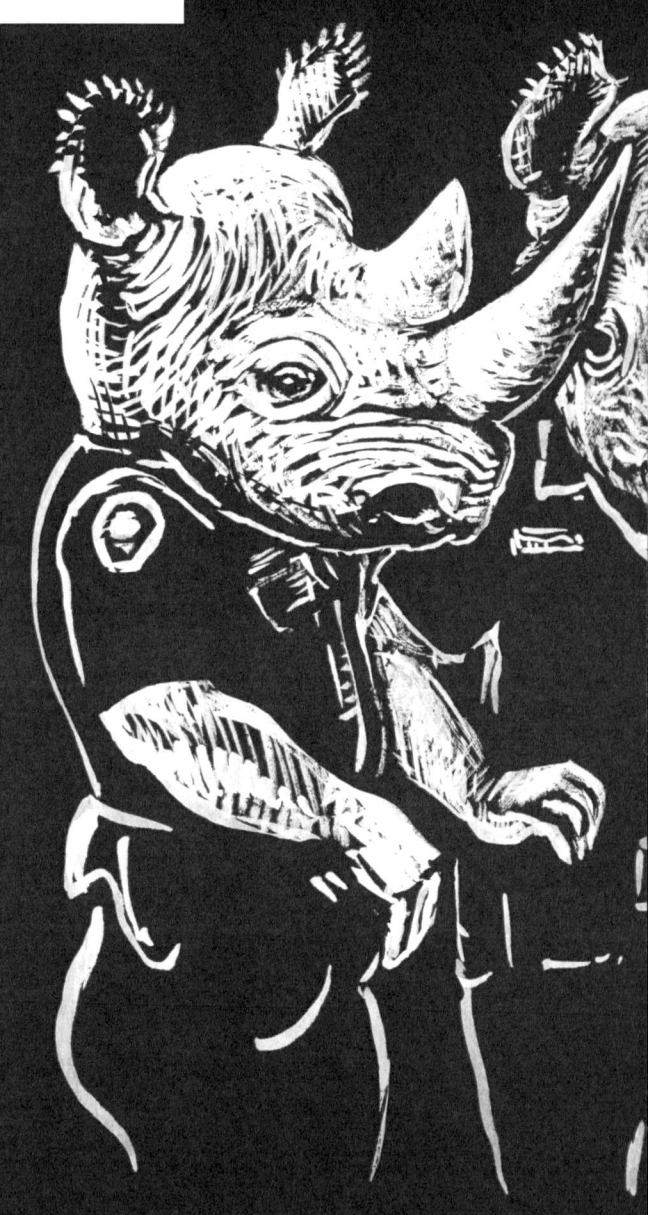

The police that responded to the domestic violence incident were useless.

They did nothing and treated me with derision.

Court ordered co-parenting counseling has not been helpful. It's an additional avenue to abuse.

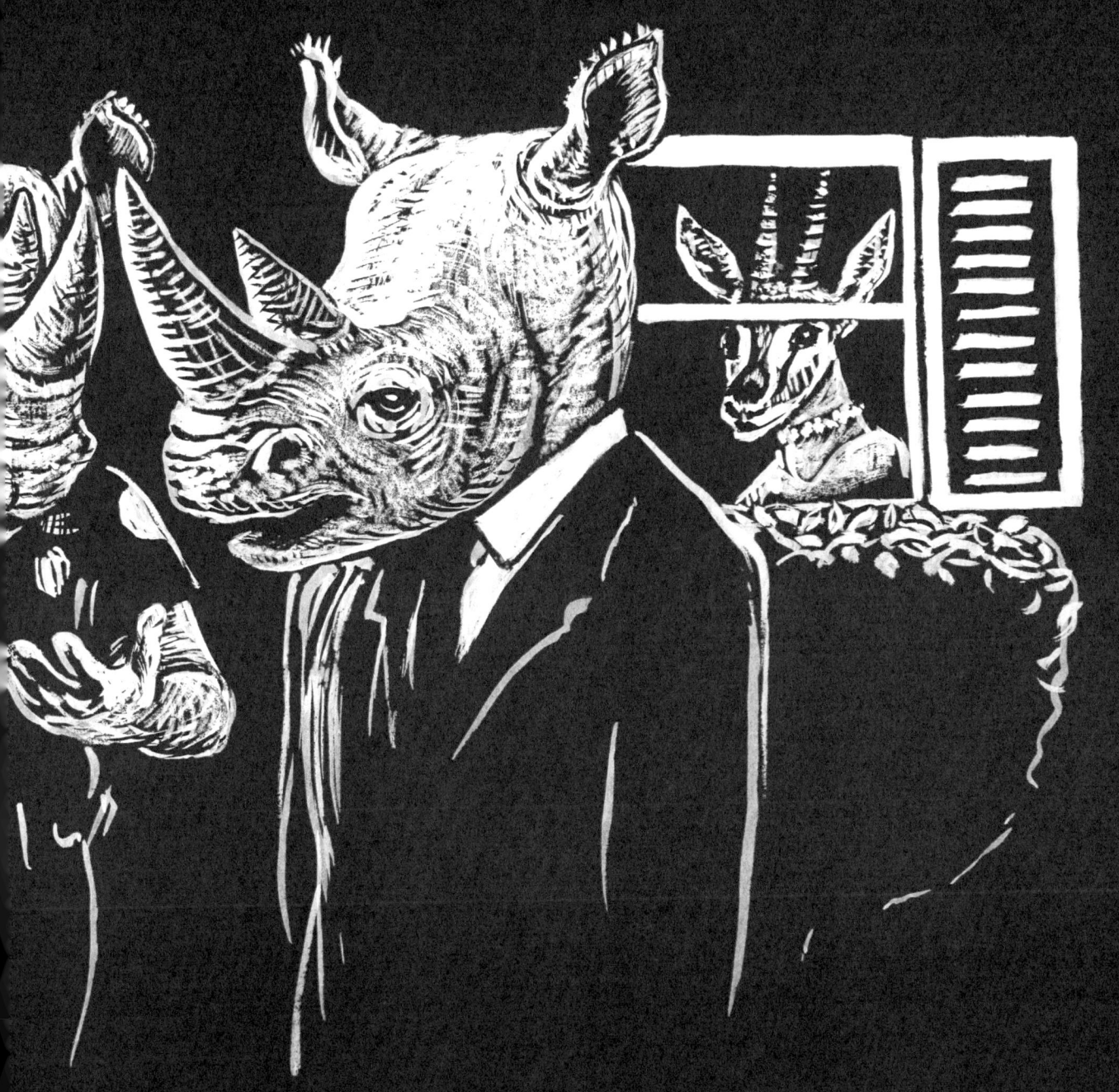

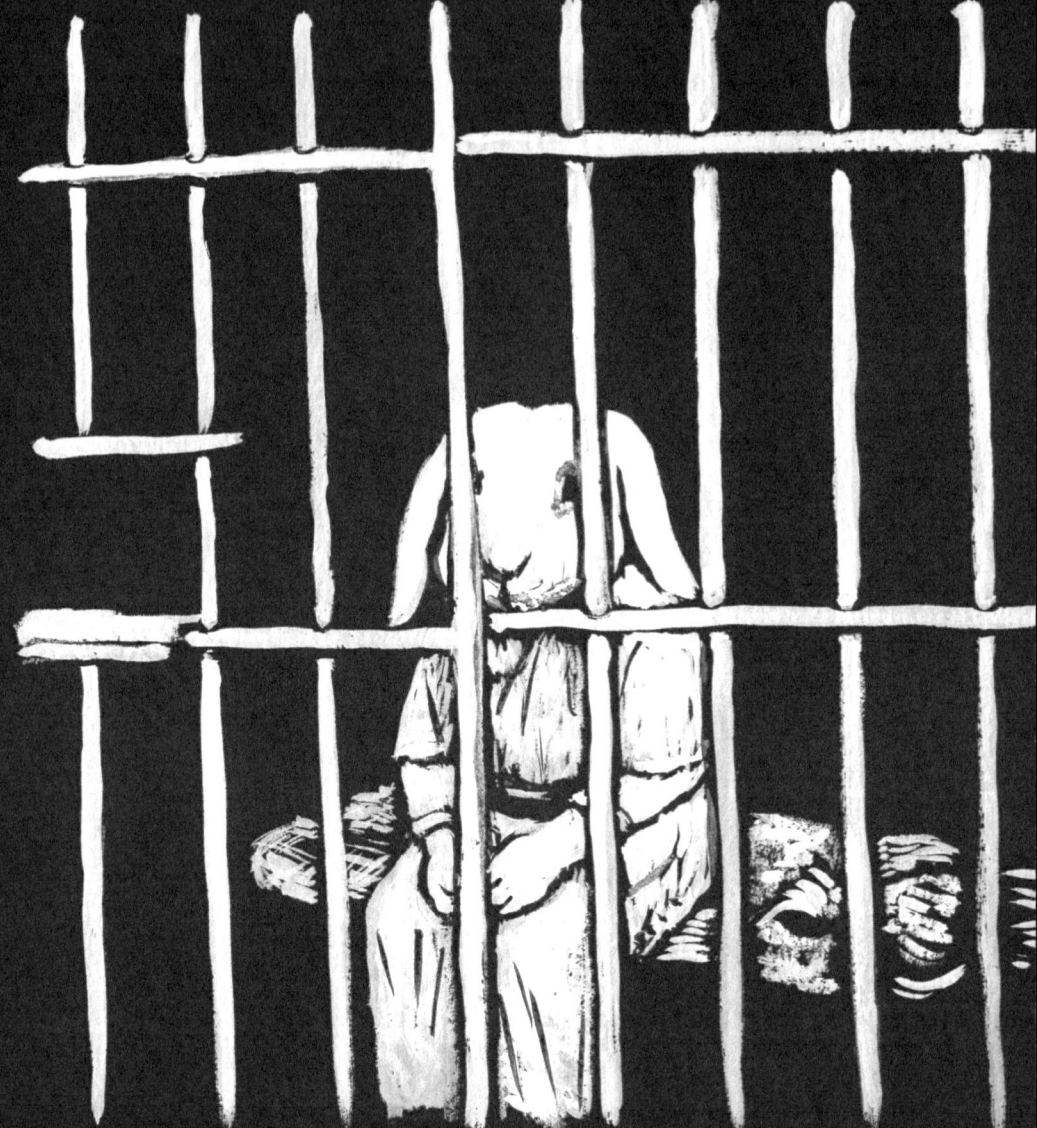

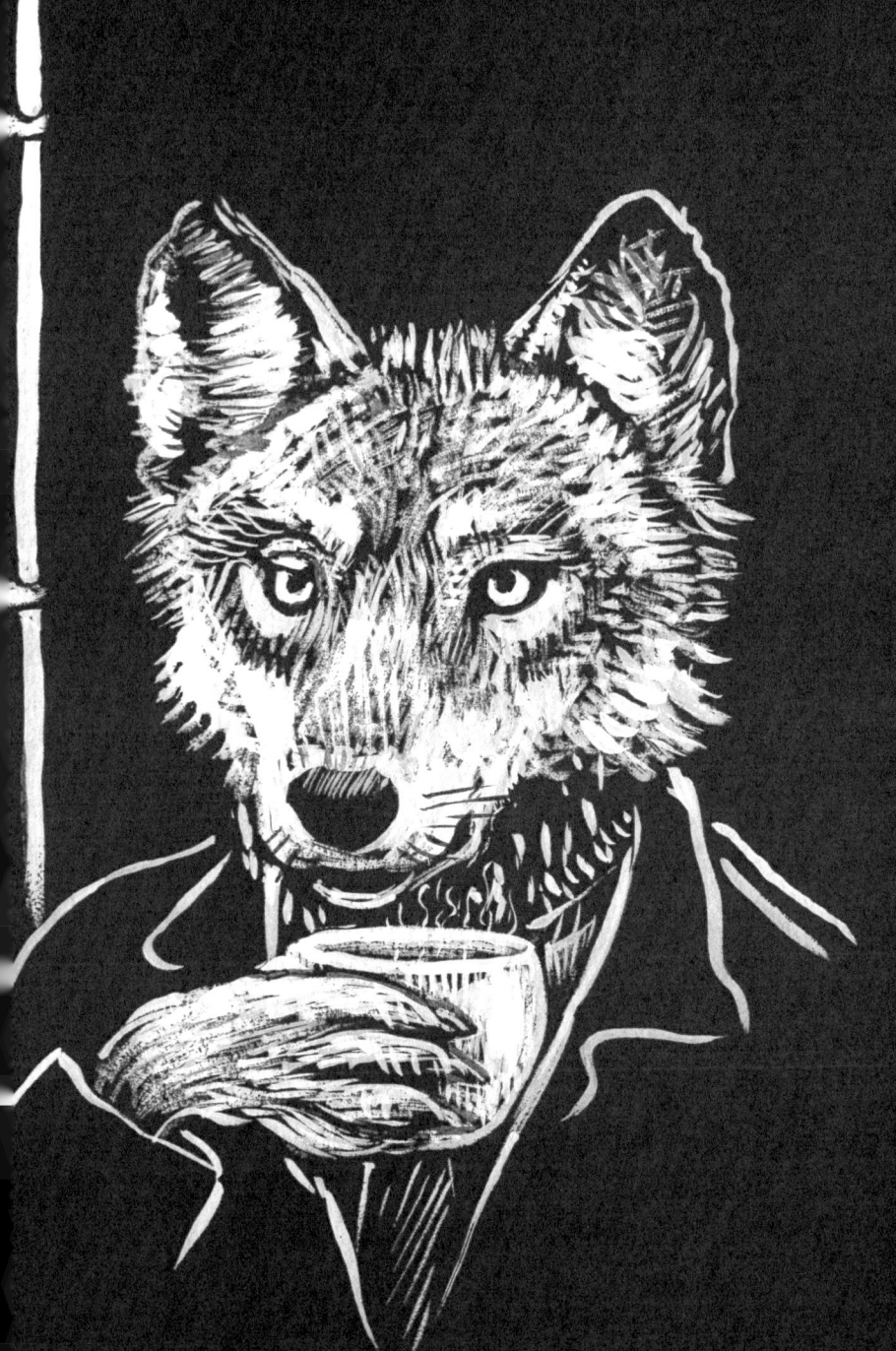

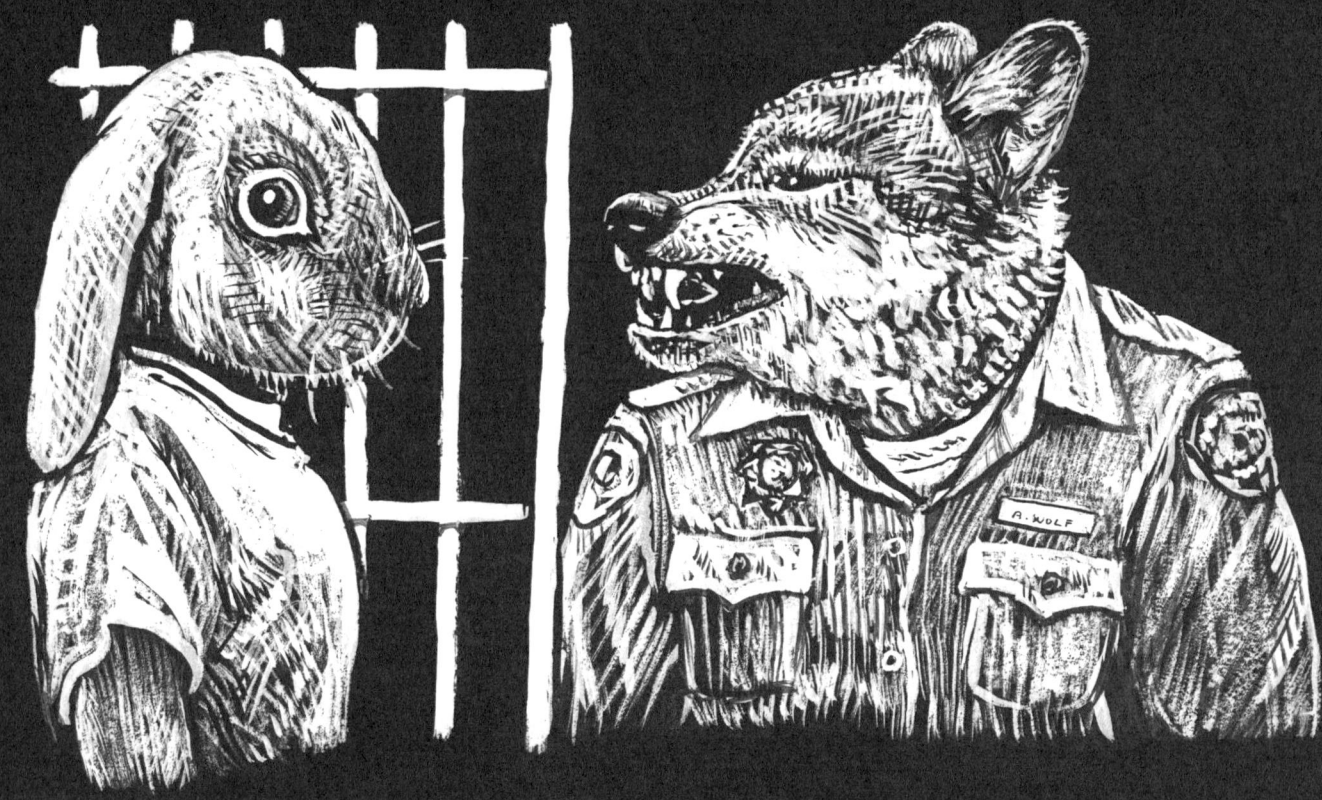

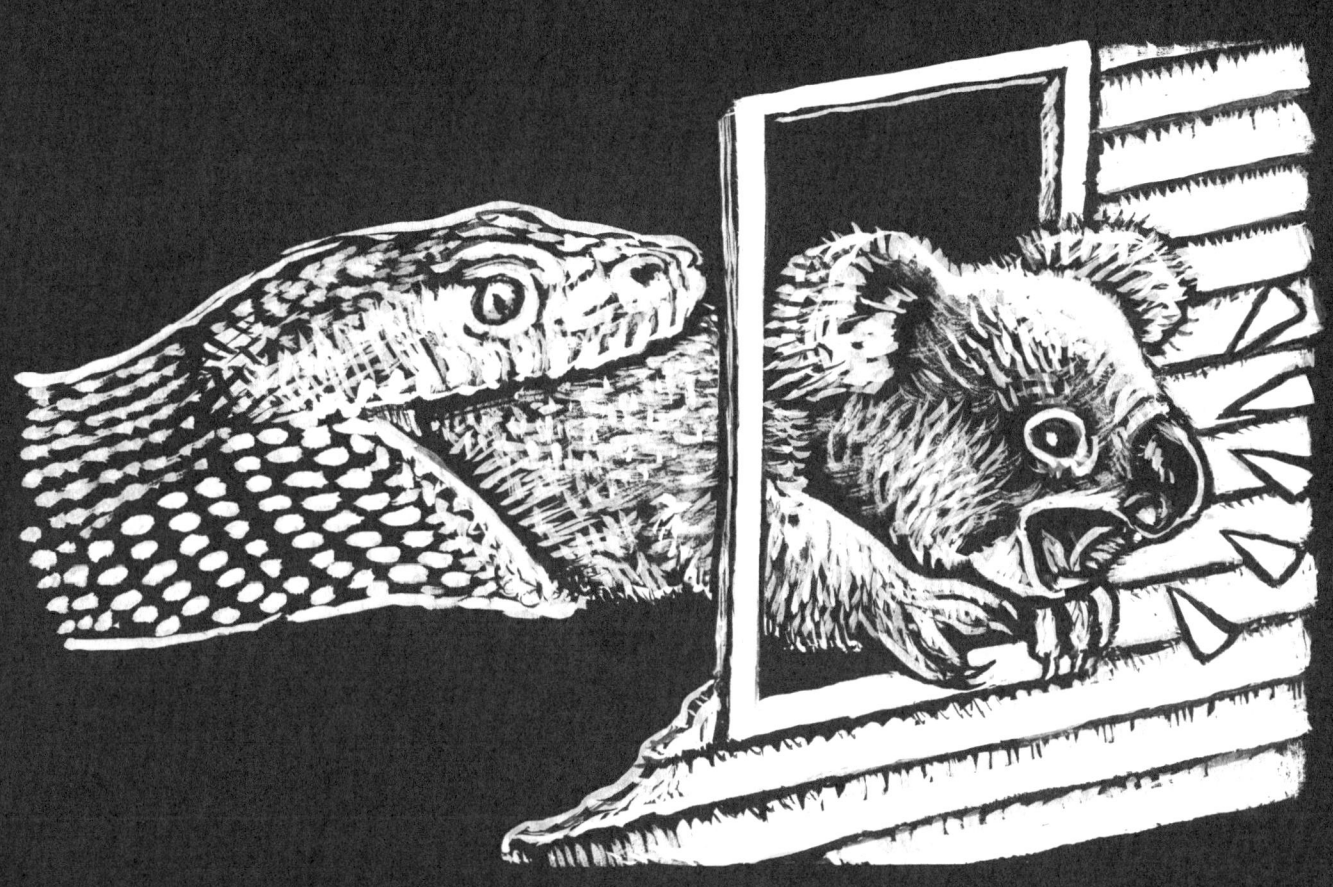

I'M AFRAID TO REPORT THE ABUSE BECAUSE I'LL BE ARRESTED AND/OR LOSE MY KIDS AND/OR BECOME HOMELESS.

- ROUGHLY 90% OF WOMEN ARRESTED FOR IPV TOWARD MEN ARE THEMSELVES VICTIMS OF VIOLENT ABUSE

- IN 29 STATES WOMEN ARE PUT IN PRISON IF THEY CAN'T STOP THEIR ABUSER FROM HARMING THEIR CHILDREN

- THE INCARCERATION RATE OF WOMEN HAS GROWN BY 834% SINCE 1978, DOUBLE THAT OF MEN

- 79% OF WOMEN IN FEDERAL AND STATE PRISONS HAVE REPORTED PAST PHYSICAL ABUSE

- 67 PERCENT OF WOMEN SENT TO PRISON IN NY IN 2005 FOR KILLING SOMEONE CLOSE TO THEM WERE ABUSED BY THAT PERSON.

- IT'S IMPOSSIBLE TO KNOW EXACTLY HOW MANY DOMESTIC VIOLENCE SURVIVORS ARE INCARCERATED NATIONWIDE FOR CRIMES DIRECTLY RELATED TO THEIR ABUSE, AS NO GOVERNMENT AGENCY GATHERS THIS DATA.

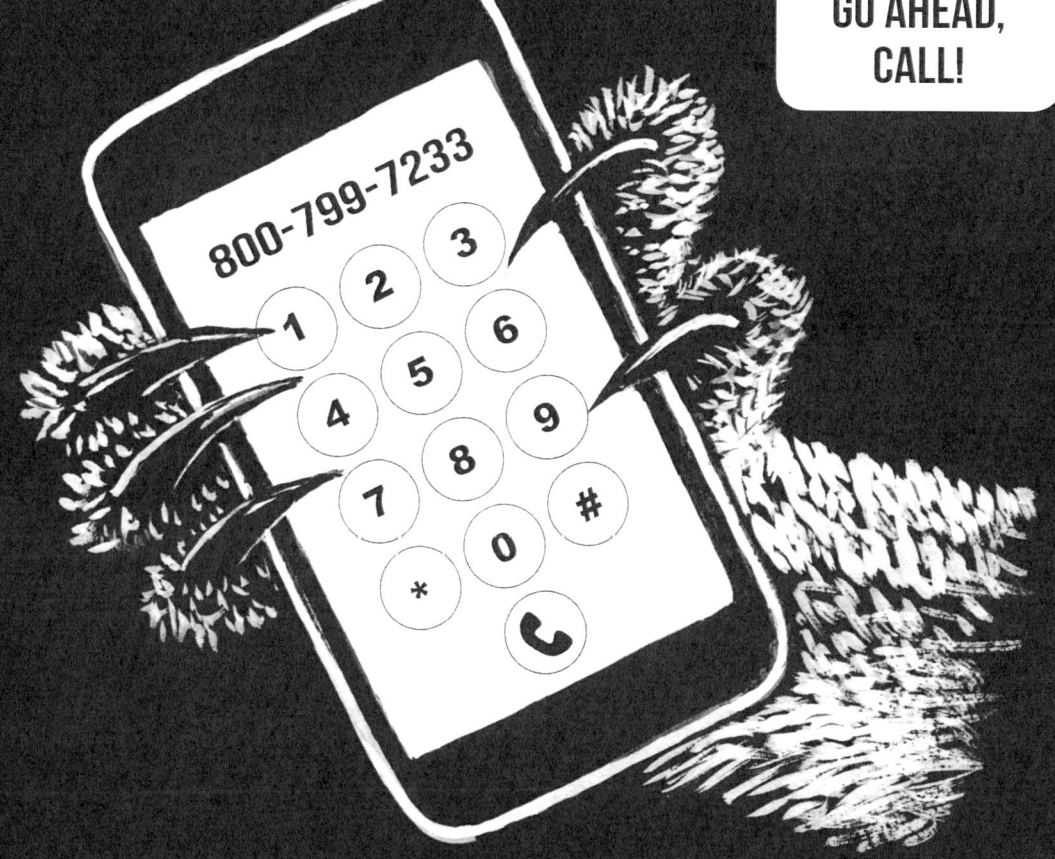

WHAT KIND OF HELP IS TRULY HELPFUL?

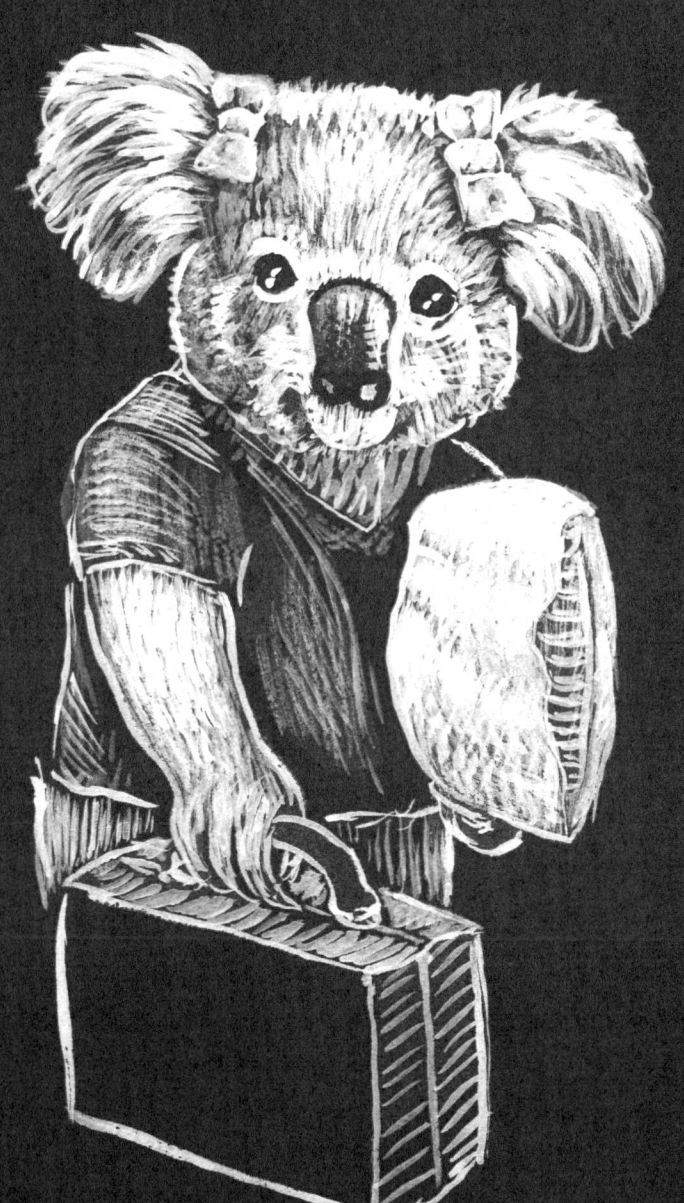

Having a place to stay ended up being the most helpful thing.

The time and space to think were critical to my recovery.

Friends helped me retrieve my belongings, and gave me a safe place to stay.

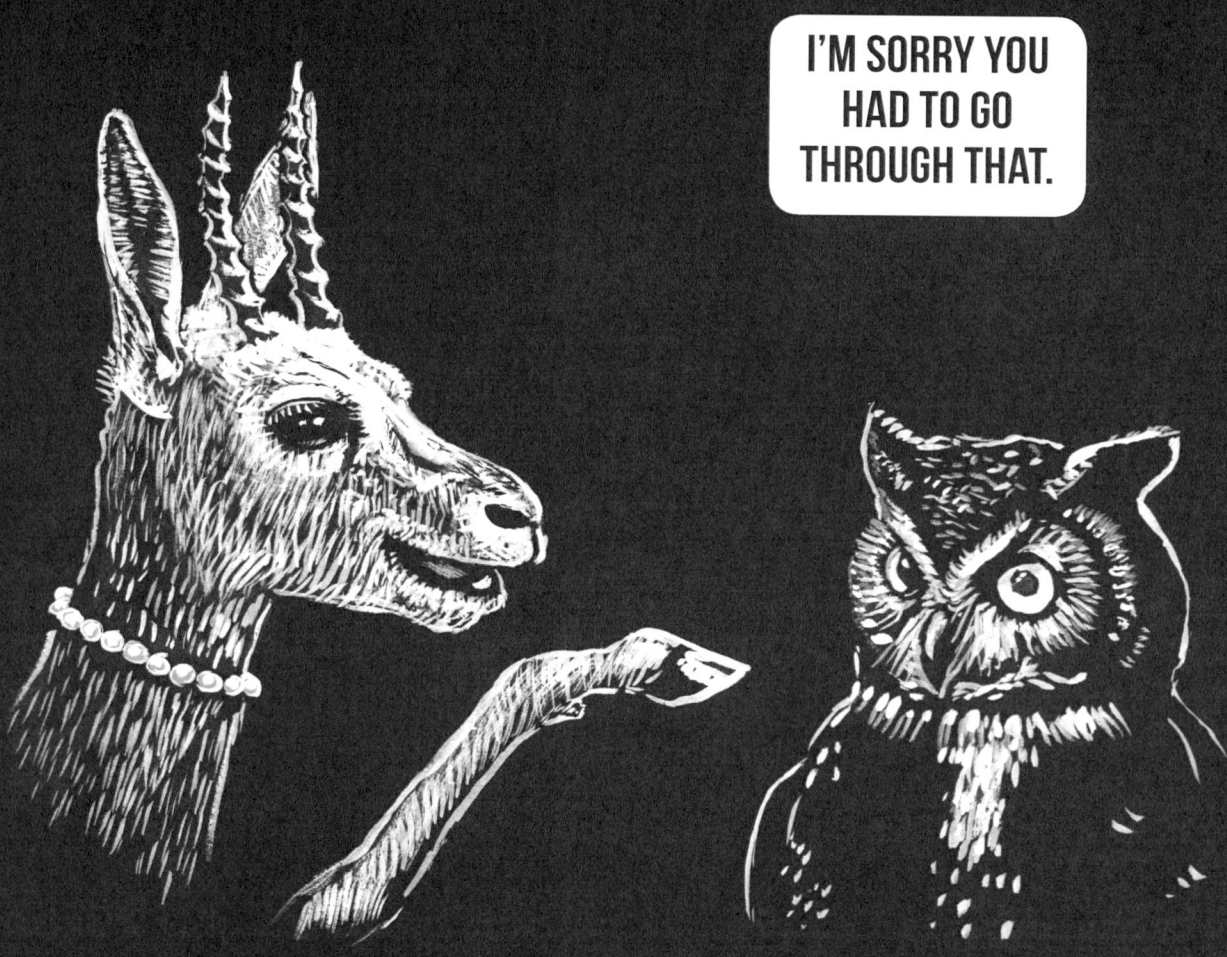

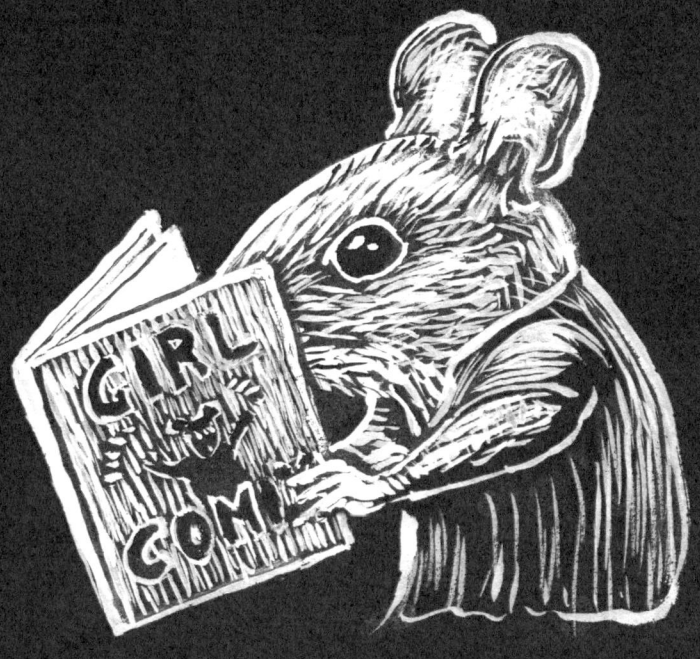

Comics were a huge thing. I read all these comics written by women, and they helped me.

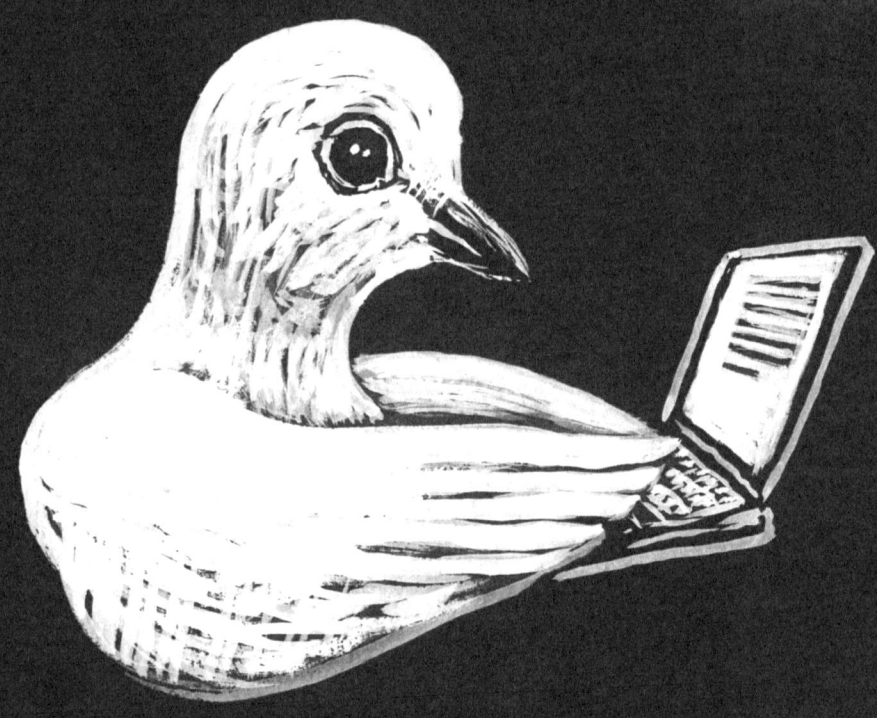

WHAT CAN I DO TO HELP MYSELF?

Just leave. Don't worry about your stuff, don't worry about your housing. Just leave and go to a shelter, or a hospital, or the police.

Write about what you're experiencing in your relationship. Going back and reading it helps to see things more clearly.

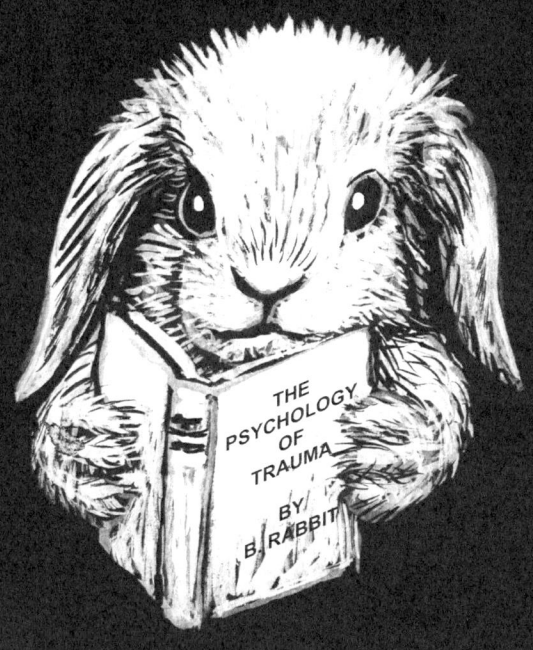

I learned so much from studying and researching the psychology of abuse.

Make plans to do things with your friends. Feel what it feels like to be accepted and treated well.

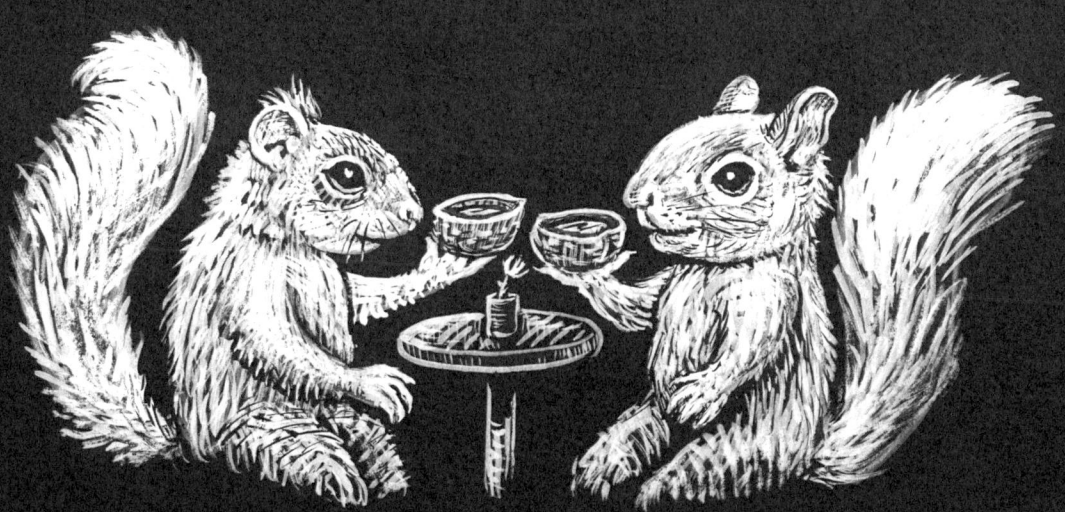

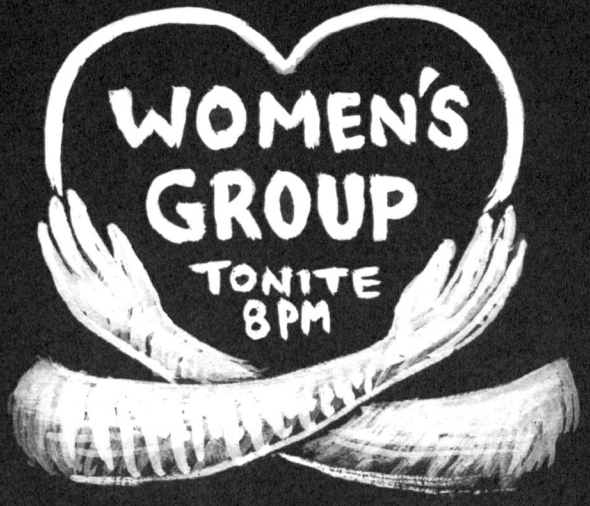

Go into physical practices: yoga, martial arts– gain ownership of your body...

Find a community, talk to someone who can validate your perceptions.

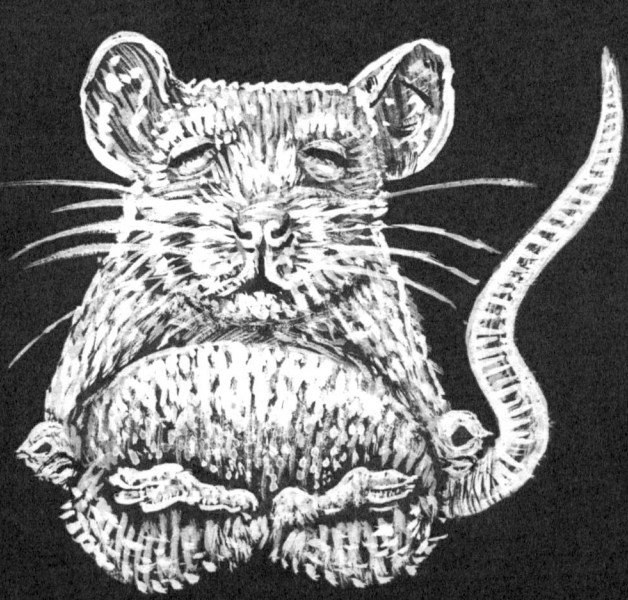

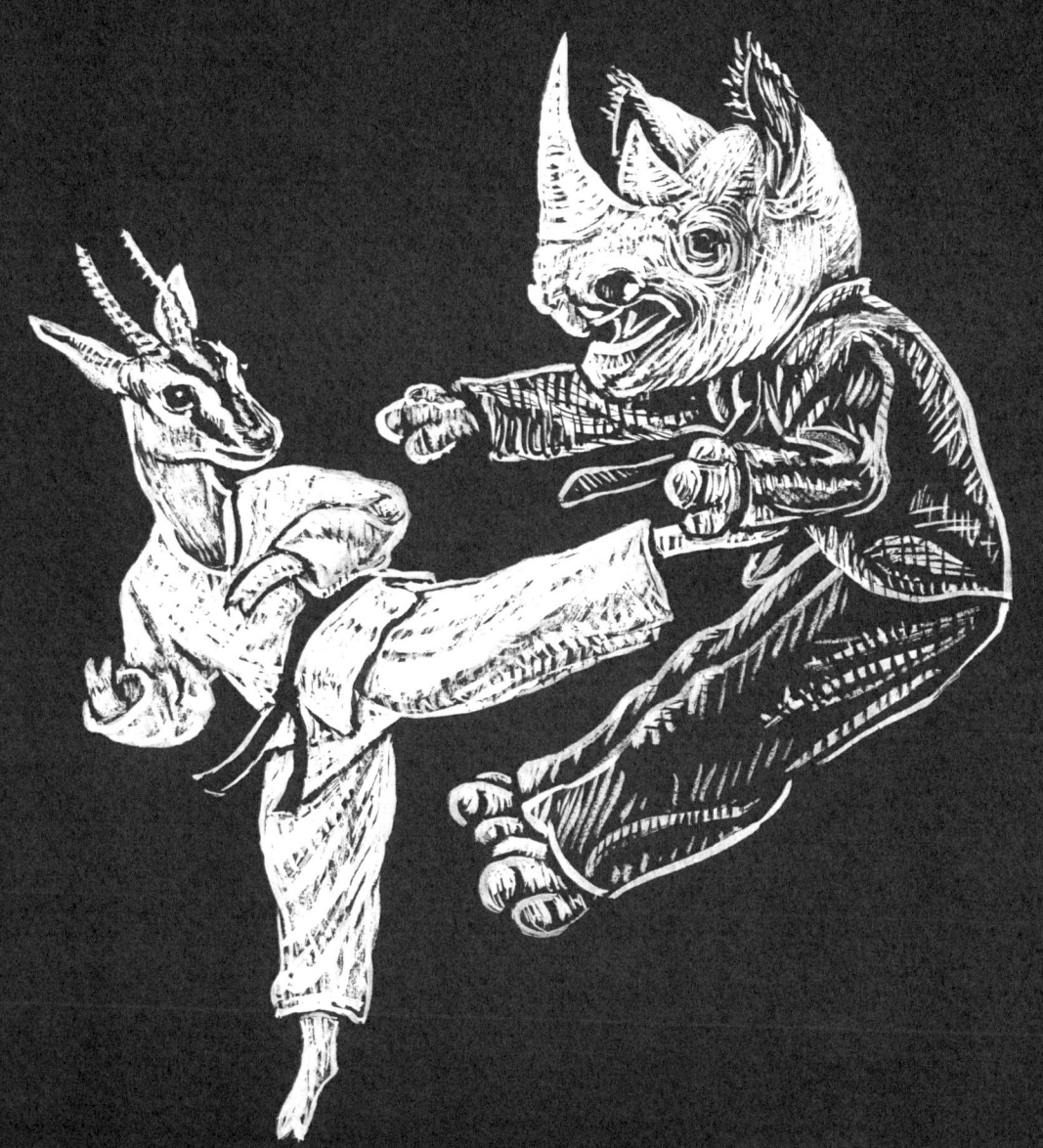

and feel your own power.

EVERY YEAR IN THE US INTIMATE PARTNER VIOLENCE:

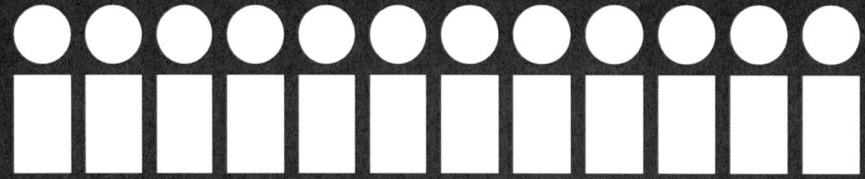

AFFECTS 12 MILLION PEOPLE

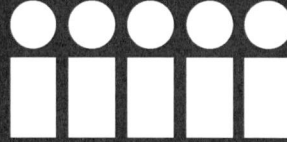

IS WITNESSED BY 5 MILLION CHILDREN

$$$$$$

COSTS VICTIMS 6 BILLION IN MEDICAL EXPENSES

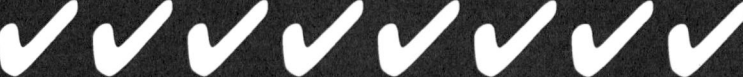

COSTS VICTIMS 8 MILLION LOST DAYS OF PAID WORK

WHAT CAN COMMUNITIES DO TO HELP?

"I wish there were more follow-ups and more support system building."

- HELP SURVIVORS FIND HOUSING, CHILDCARE AND FINANCIAL ASSISTANCE
- HOST A SURVIVORS SUPPORT GROUP AT YOUR CHURCH OR ORGANIZATION
- BUILD COMMUNITY AWARENESS ABOUT IINTIMATE PARTNER VIOLENCE

> *"I wish that we had batterer intervention programs that actually work."*

- **DEMAND LAWS THAT DON'T CRIMINALIZE SURVIVORS, OR PUT THEM OR THEIR CHILDREN AT RISK**
- **DEMAND BETTER TREATMENT OPTIONS FOR BOTH ABUSERS AND SURVIVORS**
- **DEMAND BETTER TRAINING FOR LAW ENFORCEMENT IN DEALING WITH DOMESTIC VIOLENCE**
- **DEMAND LAWS TO REMOVE FIREARMS FROM THE HANDS OF ABUSERS**
- **DEMAND THAT THE US SENATE REAUTHORIZE THE VIOLENCE AGAINST WOMEN ACT**

I THINK I'M IN AN ABUSIVE RELATIONSHIP

If your family and friends are trying to help you, let them help you. If they are not supportive, turn to your local Domestic Violence agency, or **call the national DV hotline at (800) 799-7233. DO NOT TRY TO GO IT ALONE.**

YOU ARE AT A HIGHER RISK FOR HOMICIDE IF:

- YOUR PARTNER MAKES VERBAL THREATS, ESPECIALLY THREATS OF USING A WEAPON
- YOUR PARTNER IS UNREASONABLY OR VIOLENTLY JEALOUS
- YOU ARE BEING CHOKED OR STRANGLED
- YOUR PARTNER FORCES SEX
- YOU ARE PREGNANT

If you're being abused it doesn't mean that you're stupid, and it doesn't mean that you're incapable of transformation.

It means that you're stuck in a dangerous pattern, one that you may need some help to get out of.

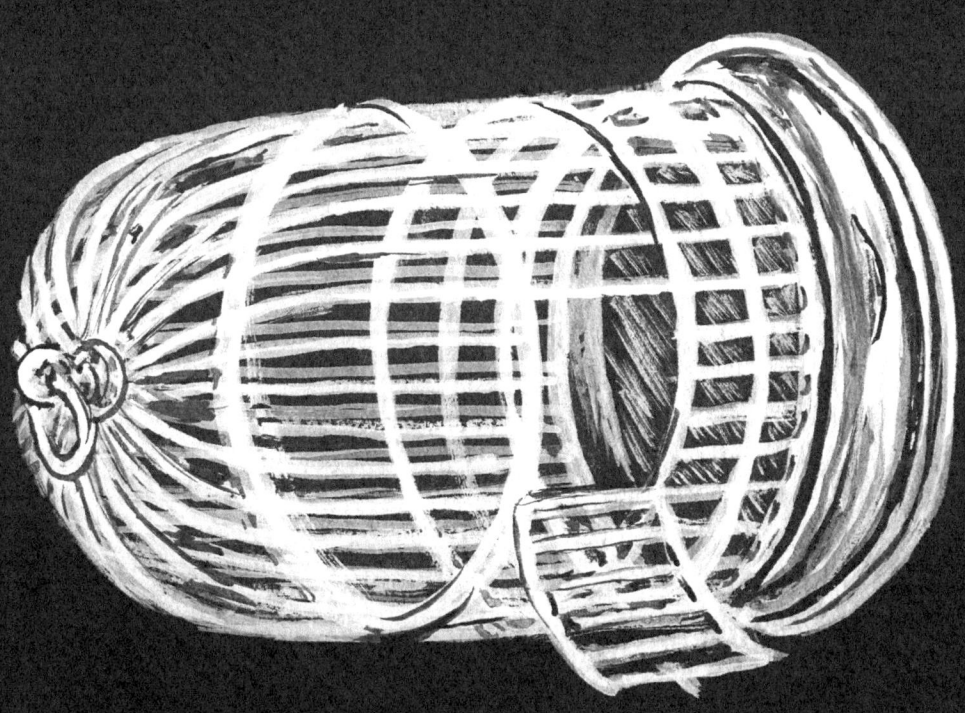

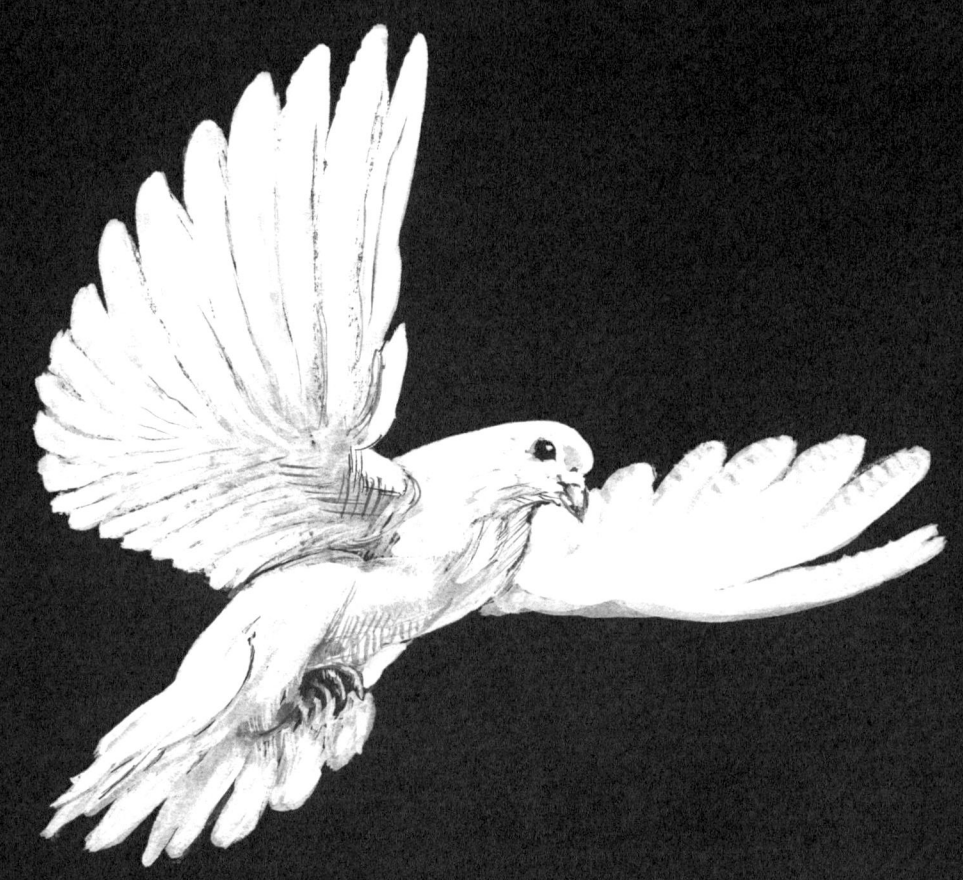

Bibliography and Sources for Statistics Cited in this Book

The National Domestic Violence Hotline

U.S. Department of Justice
"Intimate Partner Violence: Attributes of Victimization, 1993–2011"
Shannan Catalano, Ph.D

"Gender Differences in Patterns and Trends in U.S. Homicide, 1976–2017"
Emma E. Fridel and James Alan Fox

The National Coalition Against Domestic Violence

Centers for Disease Control and Prevention

Federal Bureau of Investigation (FBI)
Data analysis by AP Data Journalist Meghan Hoyer

DomesticShelters.org

childtrends.org

The Journal of Criminal Law & Criminology
"Domestic Violence and Mandatory Arrest Laws: To What Extent Do Thet Influence Police Arrest Decisions?"
David Hirschel, Eve Buzawa, April Pattavina & Don Faggiani

Violence Against Women
"When Women Tell: Intimate Partner Violence and the Factors Related to Police Notification"
Dr. Robert Peralta and Meghan Novisky

Psychology of Violence
"Gender Differences in Intimate Partner Violence Outcomes"
Jennifer E. Caldwell, Suzanne C. Swan, and V. Diane Woodbrown

"A Review of Research on Women's Use of Violence With Male Intimate Partners"
Suzanne C. Swan, PhD, Laura J. Gambone, MA, Jennifer E. Caldwell, MA, Tami P. Sullivan, PhD, and David L. Snow, PhD

Journal of Family Violence
"Gender Differences in the Impact of Family of Origin Violence on Perpetrators of Domestic Violence"
Poco Kernsmith

"Victims as Offenders: The Paradox of Women's Violence in Relationships"
Susan L. Miller. 2005. New Brunswick: Rutgers University Press

U.S. Department of Health & Human Services, Office on Women's Health
"Effects of Domestic Violence on Children"

The Crimson (Harvard University)
"When Love Hurts; How romanticizing abuse normalizes toxic and violent relationships"
Nian Hu

New York Office for the Prevention of Domestic Violence

National Clearinghouse for the Defense of Battered Women

"Should Domestic Violence Victims Go To Prison For Killing Their Abusers?: A progressive new bill in New York would give judges greater discretion when answering that question."
Melissa Jeltsen

www.ingramcontent.com/pod-product-compliance
Ingram Content Group UK Ltd.
Pitfield, Milton Keynes, MK11 3LW, UK
UKRC031943180426
11947UKWH00006B/21